Experts Agree—This Is a Must-Have Guide on Pain Management!

Just what the doctor ordered to help people with pain regain a sense of control and hopefulness about the possibilities of a satisfying and productive life.

—**Robert D. Kerns, PhD,** *Yale University, New Haven, CT*

The new gold standard for self-help books for people with chronic pain. It contains time-tested strategies designed to engage readers and bring about lasting change.

—**Robert N. Jamison, PhD,** *Professor, Harvard Medical School, Boston, MA*

This book delivers. It goes beyond pain: It's about taking control of your health, feelings, and life.

—**Akiko Okifuji, PhD,** *Professor, Division of Pain Medicine, Department of Anesthesiology, University of Utah, Salt Lake City*

The PAIN SURVIVAL GUIDE

The
PAIN
SURVIVAL
GUIDE

HOW TO BECOME
RESILIENT AND RECLAIM
YOUR LIFE

REVISED EDITION

DENNIS C. TURK, PhD
FRITS WINTER, PhD

AMERICAN PSYCHOLOGICAL ASSOCIATION
Washington, DC

Published by
APA LifeTools
750 First Street, NE
Washington, DC 20002
https://www.apa.org

Order Department
https://www.apa.org/pubs/books
order@apa.org

In the U.K., Europe, Africa, and the Middle East, copies may be ordered from Eurospan
https://www.eurospanbookstore.com/apa
info@eurospangroup.com

Typeset in Meridien and Ortodoxa by Circle Graphics, Inc., Reisterstown, MD

Printer: Sheridan Books, Chelsea, MI
Cover Designer: Naylor Design, Washington, DC

Library of Congress Cataloging-in-Publication Data

Names: Turk, Dennis C., author. | Winter, Frits, author.
Title: The pain survival guide : how to become resilient and reclaim your life /
  Dennis C. Turk and Frits Winter.
Description: Revised edition. | Washington, DC : American Psychological
  Association, [2020] | Includes bibliographical references and index.
Identifiers: LCCN 2019051147 (print) | LCCN 2019051148 (ebook) |
  ISBN 9781433831829 (paperback) | ISBN 9781433832741 (ebook)
Subjects: LCSH: Chronic pain. | Pain—Psychological aspects.
Classification: LCC RB127.T872 2020 (print) | LCC RB127 (ebook) |
  DDC 616/.0472—dc23
LC record available at https://lccn.loc.gov/2019051147
LC ebook record available at https://lccn.loc.gov/2019051148

http://dx.doi.org/10.1037/0000175-000

Printed in the United States of America
Revised edition

10 9 8 7 6 5 4 3 2 1

*To all of our patients who have taught us so much
about what it means to be a person living with pain
and not just a pain patient.*

CONTENTS

A Word Before You Get Started: How This Program Can Change Your Life   3

LESSONS

  1. Becoming Your Own Pain Management Expert   **11**

  2. Activity, Rest, and Pacing   **27**

  3. Learning to Relax   **49**

  4. Are You Always Tired? Ways to Combat Fatigue   **73**

  5. Don't Let Pain Ruin Your Relationships!   **89**

  6. Changing Behavior   **109**

  7. Changing Thoughts and Feelings   **127**

  8. Gaining Self-Confidence   **145**

  9. Putting It All Together   **161**

  10. Maintenance and Coping With Setbacks   **171**

Appendix A. Common Treatments for Chronic Pain   183

Appendix B. Additional Reading   197

Appendix C. Web and Mobile Resources for Pain   201

Appendix D. Research Supporting This Pain Management Program   207

References   215

Index   221

About the Authors   229

The
PAIN
SURVIVAL
GUIDE

A Word Before You Get Started

How This Program Can Change Your Life

If you feel pain much of the time, or if you have repeated episodes of severe pain over months or even years, you are very aware of how pain affects the quality of all parts of your life (physical, emotional, social, work, and household tasks). Only you know how your family and friends have been affected, the favorite activities you have given up, the social activities you've declined, and even the friends you have lost because of your pain-induced limitations. Perhaps you have tried medical treatments such as over-the-counter or prescription drugs, physical therapy, surgery, or complementary treatments such as chiropractic manipulations, dietary supplements, massage, or acupuncture.

Recently, the media has been filled with scary stories about one of the most commonly prescribed medications for pain—opioids. This group of drugs has been shown to be extremely beneficial for the short-term (acute) and chronic pain associated with cancer. In the past 40 years, opioids have also been prescribed for many chronic pain conditions that are not associated with cancer, in the hope that they would provide relief with limited negative effects. Only more recently have efforts been made to determine whether these drugs can be effective for controlling pain in the long term. The results have not been encouraging. Opioid drugs do not appear to demonstrate significant benefits when used on a long-term basis; moreover, they have been shown to have many negative physical and psychological effects including significant risks of dependence, misuse, abuse, and addiction (Ashburn & Fleisher, 2018; Buse et al., 2018). (Note that complete reference information for all materials cited in *The Pain Survival Guide* is included in the reference list at the end of the book.)

In addition, there is growing evidence that prescription opioids can lead to increased pain severity and, as a consequence, increased doses are needed to maintain the modest benefits provided—creating a vicious circle. Faced with this evidence, providers are being encouraged and even required to reduce the number of conditions for which they prescribe opioids and to reduce the maximum doses substantially (Dowell, Haegerich, & Chou, 2016). If you have been prescribed opioids, you should discuss your continued use and the dose with your health care provider. As with all medications that you have been prescribed, you should not try to change your use on your own. Always discuss your wishes with your health care provider before making any changes.

Unfortunately, those who reduce their opioid prescriptions often do not have good options with which to replace them (Turk, Wilson, & Cahana, 2011). We provide in Appendix A an extensive list of commonly prescribed and recommended nonopioid treatments for chronic pain. However, we will be the first to acknowledge that none of the treatments in that list, taken alone or in combination, has been proven to completely eliminate pain.

When strong medications like opioids and all the other standard treatments lead to limited benefits (and sometimes substantial risks), your health care providers may tell you, "We've done all we can; you will just have to learn to live with it." Such dismissive comments are very disheartening because you may feel you have few alternatives left. You do not want to "live with" your pain. You have been living with your pain for too long already. Rather, you want to live *without* it!

What if your practitioners told you that you can live with pain in a way that allows you to reclaim your life? That would be a different story. If they told you how you could bring quality and happiness back into your life by taking steps to take charge of your life and become resilient despite your pain, you might have realistic hope.

That is where our program begins—with the restoration of hope. By following a program that is clinically proven, you will, day by day and week by week, learn to self-manage your pain and reclaim your life. But success will depend on *you* and your efforts. This is quite a different approach from most of the treatments offered, in which you are passive and a health care provider does something to you. Each of the lessons in this book is backed by research and has been proven to help people, like you, with chronic health conditions to reduce their pain and other distressing symptoms and restore the quality of their lives.

In this book, we will help you and work with you to change your feelings of hopelessness, helplessness, and despair into realistic hope, empowerment, and resilience in the face of persistent pain and its many effects on your life. If your doctors and other health care providers have thrown up their hands and said that your case is "hopeless" or "treatment resistant" or that "you have to suffer with it," we hope to help you prove them wrong. Most important, we will help you begin to live again, despite pain! This is an important point—living again *despite pain*. Although we believe that your active involvement with the strategies and techniques described throughout this book can reduce your pain, making it more manageable, we are not suggesting that your involvement with this program will completely remove or cure your pain.

WHY NOT SEEK MORE MEDICAL TREATMENT?

When you stand in line at the supermarket and see the headlines of magazines announcing remarkable new cures for arthritis, cancer, and other pain-inducing diseases, it's hard to turn away. But when you then consider these claims next to the more obviously sensational "news" about new sightings of dead people, alien abductions, and ways to lose 25 pounds in 5 days (with no effort, of course), you may reconsider the truth of such claims.

However, when you see (or when family or friends tell you about) mainstream media describing transplants of all kinds of complex organs and new heart disease surgeries and advertisements for new drugs and devices promising relief, you may more reasonably think, "Surely there must be a new treatment for my pain. Maybe one of these will work for me. Perhaps I should see the doctor again or visit an alternative medicine healer." This is understandable. We all want to believe that when we have a problem in our lives, there is someone out there who can fix it. No one suggests that there is no hope for your car when, after you have taken it in to the mechanic, it has problems again. People tell you to take the car back to the mechanic or get a new mechanic. But if your car is overheating again and again, if you use the wrong kind gas, if your driving habits are poor, you have to change something. It may not be the mechanic. Is it possible that you have to change something in your behavior or your lifestyle?

Similarly, pain can have a profound influence on your life. Just as you have to attend to your driving behaviors to keep your vehicle in good shape, you have to adapt to new circumstances when pain forces you to pay special attention to what your body needs. What to change and how to make needed changes are quests we undertake together.

If you have seen more than two doctors who are up-to-date on recent medical advances in pain, going to a third or fourth doctor is likely to cause more frustration and feelings of hopelessness.

Over the last decade, there have, indeed, been many significant advances in medicine for some medical conditions. However, despite these developments, there is currently no treatment that can eliminate *all* pain for *all* people *all* of the time. Even the most powerful treatments (namely, opioid drugs, anticonvulsant and antidepressant medications, and surgery) typically reduce pain by no more than 30%. And even reductions at this level are only seen in fewer than half of the people who receive them. Only rarely is pain completely eliminated by any of the currently available treatments. Right now, it makes more sense to become your own pain expert and begin to manage your pain and your life.

WHEN FRIENDS AND FAMILY DON'T HELP

When you have chronic pain or frequently recurring bouts of pain, you may get the feeling that not only your doctor but also your family and closest friends do not realize what it feels like to have chronic pain 24 hours a day, 365 days a year, or to experience frequent devastating acute pain at unpredictable times and with no end in sight. Unlike when you have the flu and people can see and hear its effects, pain is maddeningly invisible to anyone else but the person afflicted. There is simply no pain thermometer that you can show to someone to prove how bad you feel, and words alone may fail to capture your experience.

Some family members or friends may subtly (or not so subtly) insinuate that you are exaggerating the extent and depth of your pain or your pain-induced limitations. The truly uninformed may suspect that you want to gain attention, elicit sympathy, avoid responsibilities, or receive disability payments. Such responses can contribute to feelings of undeserved shame. And they add to feelings of frustration, anger, and depression. It may be helpful to know that everyone feels bad when his or her concerns are not taken seriously, not just you.

SO WHAT SHOULD YOU DO NOW?

Do you remember the *Peanuts* cartoon strip in which Charlie Brown is standing on the baseball mound talking to his friend Lucy? He tells her that he is not sure whether he should play baseball that day because his arm hurts, his stomach hurts, and his back hurts. Lucy advises, unsympathetically, "Play anyway! Don't let your body push you around!"

As you will see later in this book, it is not always wise to "play anyway" or play the same way. But Lucy's other point is totally in line with our thinking. As noted earlier, we do not promise or provide a miracle cure, but we will help you learn how not to "let your body push you around." We will be your advisers, teachers, coaches, and guides, and we will help you enlist people in your life to be on your team. This will ensure that you, not your pain, is in charge of your life.

Perhaps even those people whose remarks caused feelings of shame or anger in the past will be on your team once they see that you take your pain seriously enough to make self-managing it your priority. Perhaps when they see the efforts you are making, they will finally realize that your pain is real, after all, and ask how they might best be helpful in the journey. And, even if they don't, *you* will feel better. *You* will feel realistic hope, perhaps for the first time in years. *You* will take up some of your favorite activities again. And *you* will improve the quality of your life despite pain.

Are we exaggerating? Just giving you a pep talk? You will be the ultimate judge. But we promise that we are offering you a proven program that has been used successfully with thousands of people, just like you, who also confront persistent pain. A great deal of research evidence exists to support our confidence in our approach to a wide variety of pain problems—back pain, fibromyalgia, chronic headache, arthritis, and many more. (In Appendix B we have listed other books you can consult for additional insight into the specific strategies, skills, and techniques detailed in each lesson.)

There are two things we must tell you, however. First, our program comes with a warning label. As with instructions on labels of antibiotic drugs, you must "take all the treatment in the book (bottle)" to obtain the full set of benefits. Second, although this program may appear relatively simple, simple does not necessarily mean easy. We know of no easy way to manage chronic pain. It does not exist. You will have to make pain self-management an important priority in your life. With regular and continued practice, what you learn over time will help you become more resilient and reclaim your life (but remember, despite your efforts, you should have realistic expectations about what you can achieve).

AN OVERVIEW OF THIS PROGRAM

The program we have prepared consists of 10 related lessons. Each has a specific focus, but all are designed to help you gain control of your pain and your life. In fact, if these lessons are put into practice consistently, they can help you thrive despite pain.

In Lesson 1, you will learn about pain in general and about the incapacitating effects of chronic pain. You will learn that you are not alone. Surveys have shown that up to one third of the population of the United States and worldwide have some form of chronic or recurring pain problem. Most important, you will also learn some of the erroneous and harmful myths about pain. Believing these myths as if they were facts interferes with your ability to gain control over your pain. Knowledge is the true beginning of power.

In Lesson 2, you will learn to recognize the first important pain reducer—a pattern of optimal activity, rest, and pacing. Rather than the extremes of remaining immobile or pushing yourself too hard, you will learn how to find a proper balance between activity (exertion) and rest. You will learn the importance of pacing your activities to prevent increased pain while still being able to enjoy being active and accomplishing what you need to do and find important. Practicing will enable you to gradually increase your energy, activities, and conditioning without harming yourself or making your pain worse.

In Lesson 3, you will learn to recognize the value of the second key pain reducer—relaxation. This relaxation is not the kind in which you put your feet up and watch television in a mindless haze. You're probably bored with that by now anyway, even if you may want to deny it at times. Instead, you will learn how you can create deep relaxation and achieve beneficial rest and hence enjoy many activities you may not have considered before.

In Lesson 4, we discuss the problems of chronic tiredness (fatigue) and disturbed sleep that many of our patients report experiencing. We share with you our best knowledge of how to reduce chronic fatigue and achieve a good night's rest. As you *consistently* practice Lessons 2, 3, and 4, you should notice a reduction in your experience of pain. Passively watching television will be even *more* boring because you will have better things to do with your time! Up to this point, you've been working alone with us, your guides.

In Lesson 5, you will learn how you can include other people in your life as teammates. We teach you to communicate with others in your life in such a way that they will support and encourage you. If they are stubborn, we help you find new people who can provide understanding and support and help you make the most of this program. You may not need a large team, but you do need at least one or two people to support you, encourage you, and appreciate your efforts. Understanding, acceptance, and support of others are proven pain reducers.

In Lesson 6, we focus on changing behavior—your own especially, but that of others around you as well—by applying the "laws of learning." We will teach you a number of principles with which you can influence your behavior and (sometimes) that of others. You will learn how the behaviors and responses of others affect you, even without your being aware of this. You will also learn how to change certain aspects of your lifestyle that contribute to (note that we do not say *cause*) or worsen your pain.

In Lesson 7, we focus on how you think and feel when you experience pain and its effects on your life. We know you are not creating your pain by your thoughts and emotional reactions. But you can help manage your pain by changing how you think about and react to it. You will learn how you can influence and control your mental and emotional responses to the very real pain you are experiencing. You will be able to direct your thoughts and feelings so that they contribute to your sense of control and resourcefulness rather than to feelings of helplessness, hopelessness, and despair.

In Lesson 8, you will learn to regain self-confidence and to trust yourself again. Trusting yourself may seem odd. We usually think of trust as having to do with other people. However, people with chronic pain often lose trust in their bodies and hence themselves. If others are not supportive (and we include some health care practitioners here), you may lose trust in them as well. Trust, especially in yourself, and self-confidence are potent factors in managing pain. You will learn coping skills and problem-solving strategies to regain self-trust and self-confidence. These will allow you to manage your pain further.

In Lesson 9, you will learn more about the relation between your pain and how your daily habits may be influencing your awareness of and sensitivity to pain. You will also learn how your past experiences affect your relationship with pain now. You will learn to identify and change more things in your life that are contributing to the negative effects of your pain.

If you have reached Lesson 10 and have worked at each lesson diligently, you will have become more resilient in the face of pain and be much happier, and you will have taken on many activities you never thought you would do again. However, it is just as important to learn to maintain these gains even when some level of pain continues or you have flare-ups of your pain.

In Lesson 10, we help you continue your self-management program, manage setbacks and relapses, and maintain the benefits you have achieved. As you learn that you can bounce back, you will be even more likely to confront and seek out new challenges. You will learn how to be resilient and to stay motivated for life!

In the lessons, we share several stories taken from our experience as clinicians. We have disguised the names of all individuals we discuss as examples and have taken care to change details of their cases so they cannot be identified.

We strongly encourage you to keep a diary or journal of your journey as you work through the lessons in this program. At the end of each lesson, we have included a set of questions for you to consider or exercises for you to complete. We have designed each "assignment" to help you practice specific skills and ways to manage your pain. You don't have to do all of them. However, we encourage you to try at least a few. Some of our patients tell us they have gained the most from choosing the one question or exercise that they least wanted to answer or do. Participating in this way will help you relate the information in the lesson to your unique circumstances.

Most important are our suggestions for keeping track of your progress. The charts we introduce in Lessons 2 and 3 can be photocopied and should be kept in your journal or a notebook and referred to on an ongoing basis. They may also be downloaded and printed from http://pubs.apa.org/books/supp/turk. These records are critical because improvements can be so gradual that you may not know you are improving unless you have a record to look back on. Also, you may have heard that keeping a food diary has been shown to be a, if not *the* critical component in most weight-reduction programs. The same is true for reducing pain; keeping track of your efforts (not just successes) can help you get on track and stay on track over your journey.

At the end of the book, we also include a list of suggested additional reading, organized by lesson. These readings are optional, but they may help you when your motivation is lagging. Most of the books listed can be obtained from libraries or bookstores in your community or ordered online.

A NOTE OF ENCOURAGEMENT

One of the many people who has consistently followed our pain management program wrote to us about her biggest achievement. She said,

> Before the program, I got up with the thought "Heavens, another long, painful day. I wish it were evening again." In the evening, in bed I thought, "Heavens, another long, painful night, I wish it were morning again." In my darkest hours, I even thought that perhaps it would be better if I did not see the morning again. I knew that this was not living. I didn't want to grow old like this. After consistently

following this program, I now sleep reasonably well, enjoy friends, family, and activities, and when I wake up, I look forward to the new day, even though I still have some pain.

Another reader of the first edition of this book said, "The desire to continue living and being able to feel a considerable degree of control over pain is the greatest achievement of my life, outside of raising my children."

One other reader who wrote to us noted, "I'm a new man now; I've regained my life." If you are ready to live again, and if you have opened this book, you've taken the first giant step on this journey we will take together. Let's get started.

Becoming Your Own Pain Management Expert

Grant me the serenity to accept the things I cannot change, courage to change the things I can, and wisdom to know the difference.

—SERENITY PRAYER, RHEINHOLD NEIBUHR

Everyone has pain at times—pain is important to life. It serves as a caution and a warning. The reassuring thing about most pain is that it will usually go away with time. A sports injury and its resulting pain, such as an elbow injured during a casual game of tennis, will eventually heal with resting that part of the arm. Once the pain has ceased for the weekend tennis player, the suffering is soon forgotten. It is hard to describe pain that is now gone to others and even ourselves. Think back to some painful experience you had in the past that is unrelated to your current pain. How would you describe it now? How would you explain it to others? It is hard to remember the specific feelings you were experiencing at that time.

For most people, it is unthinkable that pain will never go away. That is part of why they don't understand the plight of those who experience chronic pain. Even those with chronic pain don't like to think of it as such. If we admit to having chronic pain, it means admitting it will last a long time or perhaps will never go away at all. It's scary to think that way, and such thinking can also make the pain seem even worse.

If health care providers have been stymied and called your pain "treatment-resistant" or "chronic," you may have asked yourself, "Have the doctors and therapists been defeated by my pain?" "Have they given up on me?" "Am I destined to a life of inactivity, anger, helplessness, suffering, and despair?" These are normal but distressing thoughts, and they can be very self-defeating. We return to the role of such thoughts and ways to alter them in realistic ways and add more helpful beliefs in Lesson 7.

The good news is that many thousands of people have proved that despite the presence of pain, they do not have to give in and give up control of their lives. They have found a middle ground. They do not deny that their pain is chronic; they are facing it and confronting their pain. They have found a balance between acceptance and change. They have become wiser and resilient, despite their pain. The Serenity Prayer with which we began this lesson seems particularly applicable, especially the words *serenity*, *courage*, and most important, *wisdom*. We return to these three important words throughout this book as reminders and prompts as we move forward.

Our goal for you in this lesson is to begin to no longer think of yourself as a patient but rather as a pain self-manager. Although it may seem now that pain is holding you completely in its grip, you can find ways to overcome its debilitating effects. You can become smarter, cleverer, and wiser as you learn about your current capabilities and increase them. You will gain control over your pain and your life. As you work through this book, it will become clear to you that although others can support you, you must become your own expert on your pain and your own pain manager.

In the coming lessons, we will guide you to become that expert. You already know more than you think you do. No one knows your pain as well as you, not even the best doctors in the world. No one knows your life as well as you do. Others may say they can help you, but despite their knowledge and wish to help, they don't know your pain and your circumstances. Even if their efforts are helpful, you are at the center, and you have to be involved. You need a comprehensive plan that matches your pain and your unique situation. It is your expertise in pain that will help you design a plan based on our lessons to manage your pain, which is as unique as you are. In this lesson, you will learn more about pain so that you can better understand your own. Knowledge is power!

THE NATURE OF CHRONIC PAIN

We have used the phrase *chronic pain* several times already, but what exactly defines pain as chronic? Usually, pain following overuse or injury is considered to be chronic when it continues to interfere with living or does not become less intense after the expected period of healing—the medical estimate as to how long it takes for tissue damage to heal following that specific type of injury or overuse. Pain is also considered chronic when it is related to a progressive disease, such as arthritis or cancer.

For most acute injuries, such as a sprained ankle, the expected period of healing is from several weeks to several months. For back injuries, the pain may last longer, but with proper care, it should lessen and be completely gone over a period of time. For pain following minor surgery, the expected period of healing might only be a few days. Thus, there is no exact time at which pain ceases to be acute and becomes chronic. But most of us know when we have a chronic disease such as arthritis. We also tend to know when pain from an injury has persisted well beyond the expected course. And we can all agree that pain has become chronic when it alters our lifestyle and serves no useful purpose.

Chronic Pain Is Very Common—All Too Common!

When we have chronic pain, it is easy to feel as if we are alone. The reality is, however, that chronic pain is unfortunately very common. Recent surveys have provided some rather surprising statistics about pain. Among adults in the United States alone,

- over 10 million people report high levels of pain most days, and 8 million have pain severe enough to interfere with their lives;
- over 11 million people experience migraine headaches;
- 52 million people report the presence of chronic back pain;
- 9.2 million women report chronic pelvic pain;
- 37 million people indicate they have pain associated with arthritis;
- 3 million to 6 million people are diagnosed with fibromyalgia;
- 3.5 million people experience pain associated with cancer and its treatment; and
- annual costs (health care, disability, lost productivity) of chronic pain may exceed $600 billion.

Comparable statistics have been reported in many other countries. So, Americans are not unique when it comes to the extent and costs of pain.

Although pain is a personal experience, you have a lot of company when it comes to having chronic pain. Of course, knowing that such large numbers of others experience chronic pain does not diminish your suffering one bit and may not be all that comforting. But at least there is some comfort in knowing that you are not alone. There are many support groups consisting of others who are living with various chronic diseases and chronic pain problems. Even if your community does not have groups that meet in person or you are not able to travel to such a group, online support is often only a few Internet clicks away. Various social media groups provide numerous opportunities for you to identify, contact, and interact with others. We have included a list of some websites you might want to access in Appendix C. Depending on your interests and preferences, you might wish to reach out and interact with others who have similar problems as you. Many of these people have learned to live fulfilling lives despite their pain. They have learned to be resilient, and YOU can too!

You Can Have Harm but Feel No Pain

Acute pain can be useful as a warning that you have gone beyond your body's limitations, but the pain signaling system is unreliable at times and even deceptive. Sometimes, harm is occurring within the body and no pain is experienced. Even more often, the opposite occurs: Harm cannot be detected with standard medical tests, but pain is clearly present.

Often, people with cancer feel quite healthy until their disease progresses to a very serious condition. A lump that is not noticeable to anyone but a well-trained physician can be discovered during a routine medical checkup and turn out to be cancerous. The patient in question may feel no pain at all, and yet something life-threatening is occurring in his or her body. Following successful surgery or chemotherapy, he or she may still experience pain or other kinds of discomfort in which the pain is not caused by the tumor but by the treatment itself. For example, injuries to nerves may result from some treatments—so the original disease may be gone, but pain persists. Likewise, there are a substantial number of people who do not report pain, but when diagnostic tests such as x-rays are performed, significant pathology is present. In fact, studies have shown that when sophisticated diagnostic procedures such as magnetic resonance images (MRIs) and computerized axial tomography (CAT) scans are performed, as many as 35% of people who have no reported symptoms and no pain at all show significant physical pathology. This is pathology that we might reasonably expect to cause pain! Contrary to what we might believe, there is not a close relationship between the amount of pain we feel and the amount of damage in our bodies.

You Can Have Pain but No Detectable Evidence of Harm

There are many common chronic pain conditions, such as back pain, whiplash (resulting from neck injuries frequently following motor vehicle accidents), fibromyalgia (a painful musculoskeletal condition characterized by widespread and persistent pain and fatigue), and migraine and tension headaches, in which little evidence of physical pathology can be detected. For example, in up to 85% of people with back pain, doctors are unable to determine a physical cause. Yet, such pain may be severe, causing significant distress and disability. In the case of chronic headaches, there is rarely any identifiable tissue damage that can explain the experience of pain, yet these people suffer enormously. In whiplash injuries and fibromyalgia, no physical cause can be identified in a substantial majority of the people who report that their pain is severe and greatly diminishes the quality of their lives.

Some people for whom medical tests do not show a cause for their pain may be told outright that their pain is not real (it's all in their heads!). Or more often, they receive subtle signals from doctors, family members, or insurance and disability claims managers that they are exaggerating normal aches and pains. You may have experienced such skepticism yourself. We do not agree with such messages. All pain is real to the person who experiences it! Skepticism and disbelief are distressing and contribute to suffering on top of the pain itself.

Same Injury, Same Treatment, Different Results

Another puzzling aspect of pain is the fact that people with the same medical diagnosis of injury or disease often respond quite differently to identical treatments. For example, the majority of patients who have hip or knee replacement surgery are essentially cured, implying they should be pain free following the surgery; however, up to 20% continue to report persistent pain despite "successful surgery." Consider three people who may have surgery for a problem that is apparently caused by a dysfunction of a spinal disc (such discs function as "shock absorbers" between the vertebrae in the spine). Following surgery, one patient is happy because the pain is gone. Another is disappointed and surprised to find the pain feels the same. A third person is distressed because the pain feels even worse than before the surgery. These are common experiences for people who have undergone disc surgery. Often when this occurs, the surgeon will indicate that the surgery was performed successfully, and the damage is repaired. The results, however, suggest that factors other than damage to the disc, bones, nerves, and muscles associated with the hip, knee, or spine must be contributing to the pain experienced after surgery.

Misleading Pain

There are also a number of pain disorders in which the pain system gives a misleading signal. You feel pain in one place, but the damage is somewhere else. Doctors call this *referred pain*. The pain at one place in the body *refers* to damage somewhere else in the body. For example, pain on the side of the biceps in the arm may indicate a frozen shoulder syndrome. Back pain may be caused by problems in the stomach or pelvis. Pain radiating down the left arm may signal damage to the heart.

Finally, there are unusual pain experiences that occur following amputation or after damage to the spinal cord. Quite commonly, pain is felt as if it were in the amputated limb—a limb that is no longer attached to a body. This is referred to as *phantom limb pain*. However, whereas the limb may be a phantom, the pain certainly is not!

Pain is also frequently felt in the lower limbs of people who have had a spinal cord injury and are paralyzed. Some of these individuals experience real pain in their legs although they cannot move them. This experience of pain is surprising because through damage to the spinal cord, signals of pain do not reach the brain where pain is interpreted, and there should not be any feeling of pain. Yet, a significant proportion of people with spinal cord injuries do, in fact, feel severe pain. How can this be? It is as if the plug has been pulled from the radio, but the music is still playing. Pain is indeed one of the most mysterious of physical maladies. That is why it has been so difficult to find a cure for all sources of pain in all people.

TAKE YOUR PAIN SERIOUSLY

Extreme pain is real, even if there is no "objective" (that is, observable) cause for it as defined by current medical diagnostic techniques. The same is true for depression. A person can be depressed or suicidal when his or her whole life is going well, and nothing will show up on any medical test. And this has been true since time immemorial, but only in the past few decades has the medical establishment acknowledged it. The Russian author Leo Tolstoy once wrote, "I am very rich and famous; millions of Russians read my books. I possess a big farm, a wife, and five children, and the only thought that haunts me is: shall I use a rope or a gun to end it all?"

Many people with chronic pain become depressed. If this is true for you, then we encourage you to take your depression as seriously as you take your pain and consider consulting a mental health professional to support you in your journey toward a better quality of life.

The same is true with anxiety. A person in no objective danger can break out in a sweat and feel as if he or she is going to die. That is why it is good to repeat once again that feelings of fear, sadness, and pain can be extremely intense, even if they seem out of proportion to the so-called objective facts. When belittling themselves for having pain and thinking of themselves as weak, individuals with anxiety or depression often think they are "going crazy."

Neither the person experiencing unremitting pain nor the person experiencing anxiety or depression is weak or crazy. What they have in common is that they must search for a solution (or solutions) that can improve their lives rather than focusing on what may or may not be the cause.

Seek the Solution, Not the Cause

In cases of chronic pain, both you and your health care providers initially seek to find the cause of your pain. By this, doctors usually mean the physical cause. Long after a second opinion has been sought and the doctors have "given up," you may continue to try to find the cause of the pain. However, the main issue is not how or why you got the pain. The critical issue is what you can do to manage your pain so you can get on with your life. Likewise,

- The question is not: What is the cause of the pain?
- The question is: What factors influence the pain?
- The question is not: What can the medical profession do?
- The question is: What can I do?

Later in this book, we discuss the role of pain-influencing factors other than physical damage. Here, we discuss some of them briefly in the context of the gate-control theory of pain and how this can help you understand and make sense of pain.

Gate-Control Theory of Pain

Imagine a door or gate in your spinal column. Before your pain became chronic or before you had a progressive disease such as arthritis, this gate was usually closed, and you did not feel pain. If you had an injury or some other type of obvious physical damage occurred, signals were sent along your nerves (the wiring of our bodies) to the spinal cord. These signals "opened" the gate and allowed information about the injury or damage to your body to reach the brain. This is where these signals are interpreted, with the result being the feeling of pain. In these cases, as you healed, the pain was sometimes better, and sometimes it was worse. It depended on how far open or closed the gate was.

It is important to note that regardless of where an injury occurs in the body, pain is not experienced until signals reach the brain, where perception takes place. Think of a patient who is anesthetized during surgery. The surgeon makes an incision that causes tissue damage that can be extensive, depending on the type of surgery. The question is, does the unconscious patient feel any pain? The miracle of anesthesia is that the patient does not experience pain while he or she is anesthetized. Before the discovery of anesthesia, patients exposed to surgery experienced severe pain. Anesthetic agents block the patient from perceiving the signals from the incision.

In Figure 1.1 we have included a summary of the different factors that are known to open and close the pain gate—those things that can make pain worse and those that can reduce or eliminate how we experience it.

The idea of a pain gate that can be opened and closed will help you understand that pain, especially chronic pain, cannot simply be eliminated by cutting out a painful body part or cutting nerves. In the past, nerves were cut in the hope of blocking pain. Unfortunately, all too often, the surgical procedures created more problems than they solved. The nervous system does not operate like a simple cable system that can just be clipped and repaired. It is a living, interconnected system that is continually changing and adapting to new circumstances and new information.

COMMON MYTHS ABOUT PAIN

In addition to the idea of the pain gate, it's also helpful to know that much of the common folklore about pain can actually decrease your chances of living a zestful life. We have already briefly discussed a couple of these ideas, but the information is so important to your recovery that it bears repeating.

Myth 1: Pain Is Always a Reliable Signal of Physical Damage and Injury

Pain may be a clear and reliable signal of damage to the body. When this occurs, pain is useful; it has a purpose—namely, protection. Pain makes it clear to you when the water in a bath is too hot; this information can prevent you from burning yourself. Pain makes you feel uncomfortable when you are trying on shoes that are too tight. The pain tells you not to buy them!

However, as discussed earlier, pain is not always a reliable indicator of where and to what extent harm is occurring in the body. Most important, when you have chronic pain, feeling discomfort on exertion is not necessarily an indicator for action or inaction. We talk more about this important topic in the next lesson.

FIGURE 1.1. Factors That Can Open and Close the Pain Gate

Factors that can open the pain gate

- Physical factors
    - ↑ Extent of injury
    - ↑ Inappropriate activity level

- Emotional stress
    - ↑ Depression
    - ↑ Worry or fear
    - ↑ Tension
    - ↑ Anger

- Thoughts
    - ↑ Focusing on the pain
    - ↑ Boredom due to minimal involvement in life activities
    - ↑ Nonadaptive attitudes and expectations ("It will never end!" "I'm helpless and hopeless!")

Factors that can close the pain gate

- Physical factors
    - ↓ Medication
    - ↓ Counterstimulation (heat, rubbing)
    - ↓ Appropriate activity level
    - ↓ Rest

- Relative emotional stability
    - ↓ Relaxation
    - ↓ Positive emotions (happiness, optimism)

- Thoughts
    - ↓ Life involvement, increased interest in life activities
    - ↓ Concentration or distraction
    - ↓ Adaptive attitudes or positive thoughts and feelings ("I can control my feelings," "I can reduce my level of muscle tension," "I am capable of doing many things despite my pain")

Myth 2: When No Clear Physical Damage Is Found by Diagnostic Procedures, Pain Must Be Imaginary

If this were true, millions of people with back pain, headache, phantom limb pain, and pain following spinal cord injuries would all be experiencing imaginary pain! An epidemic of imaginary pain is not very likely. The absence of identifiable physical pathology does not negate pain and related suffering, nor does it guarantee that zero physical factors are contributing to the pain. As noted earlier, all pain is real, and your pain is real, regardless of what anyone else has told you.

Myth 3: Chronic Pain That Does Not Respond to Standard Treatment Should Not Be Taken Seriously

For too long, only when a direct relationship could be found between pain and visible damage was pain taken seriously. Lack of knowledge and ignorance about chronic pain have caused great physical and emotional distress (anxiety, depression, frustration, anger) for many people. Too many individuals still believe that you can only have pain and feel pain when your pain has been legitimized by a physician who has examined you and run diagnostic tests. This implies that only a doctor can determine whether you have a right to your feelings of pain. No one has a right to tell you what you are feeling, no matter how many academic degrees he or she may have or how long he or she has been a health care provider. Unfortunately, pain is not directly observable. It is an intensely personal experience. There is, as yet, no pain thermometer that measures the internal experience of pain. Only *you* know how much pain you feel and how often you feel it.

Myth 4: There Is a Pill for Every Ill. When in Doubt, Cut It Out

People, particularly those in the United States, have been flooded with advertisements suggesting that there should be a "pill" for every problem. There are even pills for problems we didn't know we had or did not view as problems. Our media reinforce this: "Can't sleep at night? Take a pill. Don't have enough energy? Take a pill. Feel upset? Take a pill. Prevent indigestion before eating a spicy meal. Take a pill." They don't, however, tell you to change the behavior that might be contributing to the symptoms.

Surgery, too, is being recommended like never before. If you don't like the way your face or body looks, have surgery. Think you look too fat? Have liposuction. Don't like your lips? Have collagen injections. Breasts too small or too large? Implants and breast reduction surgery to the rescue! Even people with well-earned wrinkles are advised to have Botox treatments to eliminate them.

Depending on pills, surgery, and other "magical" cures sounds so much easier than learning what it takes to change your behavior or your mindset. We are not suggesting that medication and surgery are never appropriate. There are a time and place for medication and surgery. But the mass media are not qualified to make these decisions. Don't be brainwashed by their messages. Product companies and drug companies have ulterior motives for their claims—namely, to increase sales.

When it comes to pain, be informed. For example, every month there seems to be a new arthritis pill advertised on television with testimonials you can view on the Internet. Some of these are just a variation on a medication whose patent has just expired. Drug companies are given patents and exclusive rights for a limited time for their products, and after that period, often 7 years, generic products can come to market at much lower costs. What these advertisements don't tell you is that even the most potent pain medications produce only about a 35% reduction of pain and in only about half the people who take them (Turk, Wilson, & Cahana, 2011). (Note that complete reference information for all materials cited in *The Pain Survival Guide* is included in the reference list in Appendix D at the end of the book.) And taking medication definitely does not ensure long-term improvements in quality of life.

Myth 5: Pain Is a Signal to Stop Moving

In instances of pain following an acute injury or trauma (for example, a broken leg as a result of a fall from a ladder), it may be appropriate to desist from activities that increase pain. In these cases, the pain is serving as a reliable warning signal. Remember the joke about the man who goes to a doctor and says, "Doc, it hurts when I do this," and the doctor replies, "Then don't do that!"?

However, for people with chronic pain, feeling pain or discomfort with exertion is not a reliable signal to cease activity. In fact, some forms of inactivity can increase your pain (more about this later). Consider that even following heart surgery, doctors recommend certain activities because being active tends to speed recovery—although it hurts at first! The same is true for hip and knee replacements; activity is recommended as soon as possible following the surgery (often 1 day or even less). We are sure that if you ask most patients how happy they are to begin exercise soon after their surgery, they would not be very positive. They would admit it takes considerable prodding to get them moving again.

For those with chronic pain, discomfort following reasonable activities may have little to do with the original cause of the pain and more to do with the reduction in strength, endurance, and flexibility of muscles due to lack of use. These muscle changes can occur quickly with inactivity—in weeks or even a few days. In the next lesson, we describe guidelines for how to increase activity to eventually decrease pain. But for now, keep in mind that not moving may be increasing your pain and disability over time.

Myth 6: If You Have Had Pain for a Long Time and Doctors Have Told You That They Have Done All They Can, Your Situation Is Hopeless

This is perhaps the most dangerous myth we have described. It undermines your efforts to gain control over your pain and your life. As we demonstrate in this book, everyone can make changes that lead to pain reduction and improved quality of life, but acceptance, courage, action, and wisdom are required.

The traditional biomedical approach may be appropriate for acute physical problems. For example, the use of analgesic medication to control pain following major surgery is appropriate. Likewise, analgesics are appropriate when you sustain a traumatic injury like a broken bone in your arm or leg. In these instances, using analgesic medication to reduce pain and setting the bone and keeping it immobile with a cast is appropriate. However, when pain persists, and it becomes chronic, these approaches may not be best and may actually be detrimental. Medication to control pain, even if it can reduce it somewhat, is not a cure. If you have chronic pain, you will have to find a way to live effectively despite the presence of pain. Moreover, immobilization to protect a broken bone is the appropriate treatment to prevent further injury and promote healing. But over the long term, lack of use of the muscles leads to weakening from disuse and reduces functioning, fostering disability.

In Appendix A, we present an alphabetical list of common treatments and therapeutic approaches for chronic pain. The list might seem quite overwhelming. How can you decide what is best for you? The reality is that we cannot tell you. For many of the treatments and approaches listed, the benefits are rather modest. What we do know is that none of them will eliminate all your pain, and thus, regardless of the good effects, you will likely continue to have some pain. Continued dependence on others or on therapies and medication to control your pain will only lead to greater frustration if you are not actively involved in learning what works for you. Remember that, ultimately, the goal is to develop resilience and learn how best to cope despite some level of pain.

With this lesson, you have begun the journey toward a new life by becoming better informed about pain. With knowledge and, most important, application of this knowledge, you will find ways to manage your pain, be resilient, and enjoy your life again. You must put into action what you learn in each lesson.

In the next lesson, the application of knowledge begins. You will learn how to use one of the most important tools in managing your pain—activity pacing. At the end of this lesson and in all of the following lessons, we raise important questions for you to consider and suggest activities that can help you understand and manage your pain.

SUMMARY

- When you have chronic pain, life seems to have lost its purpose. Being advised that "you must learn to live with your pain" feels like a betrayal. It is only when you can give purpose and quality to your life that there is a chance you can not only live with the pain but also actually thrive, despite the pain.

- It seems unbelievable that your pain could be incurable, given the current state of modern medical knowledge. When you feel pain that persists, it is easy to feel as if you are alone. The reality is that chronic pain is very common. Huge numbers, however, do not diminish the suffering you experience.

- Contrary to what most people think, pain is not always a useful warning. The pain signaling system is often unreliable and may be disrupted. In many cases, the pain signal is anything but clear. There are a number of other myths about chronic pain that are also erroneous and harmful.

- The gate-control theory of pain explains many of the puzzles of pain—pain without physical damage, physical damage without pain. This model suggests that there is a gate that determines whether signals indicating pain reach the brain. Feelings and attention, or other factors, can open or close the "pain gate." You can learn ways to close the gate.

- Pain always has something to say, and for this reason, should always be taken seriously. Feelings such as fear, sadness, and pain can get out of control. Ignoring or denying them does not help.

- It is helpful to look for the solution to, not the cause of your pain.

- You can become your own pain self-manager. You know the pain you feel, you have your own experiences with your pain, you know your circumstances, and you need all that knowledge for designing a good plan for you.

- What you also need is information and insight into the principles that make up a successful treatment program that will help you manage your pain and limitations and regain control of your life.

QUESTIONS TO CONSIDER

In this section, we raise a number of questions. The answers you give will help you learn more about your pain and the impact the pain has on your life.

Think about each of the following questions and respond to them. (You can, of course, return to any part of the lesson if you need some help.)

1. Which of the pain myths have you heard or been led to believe? Which have you come to accept?

2. Why is the gate-control theory important for understanding chronic pain?

3. List the factors that can open your "pain gate."

4. List the factors that can close your "pain gate."

5. How predictable is your pain? Is there any pattern you can identify for the increases and decreases in your pain (for example, times of the day, following certain activities, when you get upset)?

6. What do you want to achieve with this self-management program? What goals do you have? Be specific. For example, you might have a goal of spending more time in your garden, walking in a shopping mall, or spending time with your family or friends.

HOME ACTIVITIES

1. Describe your pain (how long you have had it, where it is located, how it has changed over time).

2. List the areas of your life that have been affected by pain. What has the pain cost you? How has the pain affected your work, play, and performance in other activities? How has the pain affected your relationships with family and friends?

3. Make a list of the things you CAN do despite your pain.

4. Circle the things that make your pain WORSE.
   – Weather
   – Exercise
   – Stress
   – Cold
   – Heat
   – Arguments
   – Fatigue
   – Poor sleep
   – Depression
   – Other _____
   – Other _____
   – Other _____

5. Circle the things that make your pain BETTER.
   – Rest
   – Warm bath
   – Relaxation
   – Sleep
   – Medication
   – Exercise
   – Other _____
   – Other _____
   – Other _____

The responses to this set of questions will allow you to understand more about your pain and how it affects your life.

PAIN SELF-ASSESSMENT

We will ask you to repeat your responses to these questions several times throughout this book. At the end of the program, you will be able to see how much progress you have made. So, please do your best to respond to each question based on how you feel right now. Do not return to the responses you give until we ask you to later in the book.

1. Rate the level of your pain at the **PRESENT MOMENT**.

$$0 \quad 1 \quad 2 \quad 3 \quad 4 \quad 5 \quad 6$$

No pain   Very intense pain

2. On average, how severe has your pain been during the **PAST WEEK**?

$$0 \quad 1 \quad 2 \quad 3 \quad 4 \quad 5 \quad 6$$

Not severe   Extremely severe

3. In general, during the **PAST WEEK**, how much did your pain interfere with daily activities?

$$0 \quad 1 \quad 2 \quad 3 \quad 4 \quad 5 \quad 6$$

No interference   Extreme interference

4. During the **PAST WEEK**, how much has your pain changed the amount of satisfaction or enjoyment you get from taking part in social and recreational activities?

$$0 \quad 1 \quad 2 \quad 3 \quad 4 \quad 5 \quad 6$$

No change   Extreme change

5. During the **PAST WEEK**, how well do you feel that you have been able to deal with your problems?

$$0 \quad 1 \quad 2 \quad 3 \quad 4 \quad 5 \quad 6$$

Not at all   Extremely well

6. During the **PAST WEEK**, how successful were you in coping with stressful situations in your life?

$$0 \quad 1 \quad 2 \quad 3 \quad 4 \quad 5 \quad 6$$

Not successful   Extremely successful

Some of these questions can also be found on the West Haven-Yale Multidimensional Pain Inventory (Kerns, Turk, & Rudy, 1985).

7. During the **PAST WEEK**, how irritable have you been?

0   1   2   3   4   5   6

Not irritable   Extremely irritable

8. During the **PAST WEEK**, how tense or anxious have you been?

0   1   2   3   4   5   6

Not anxious or tense   Extremely anxious or tense

Remember, we will ask you to repeat this several times, and when you have finished Lesson 10, it will be of interest to you to see the difference between the scores now and those at the end of this book. They will also guide you back to the different lessons that were related to the focus of each question.

Activity, Rest, and Pacing

Small steps may appear unimpressive, but don't be deceived. They are the means by which perspectives are subtly altered, mountains are gradually scaled, and lives are drastically changed.

—RICHELLE E. GOODRICH, *MAKING WISHES*

One of the most frustrating things about pain is that it interferes with your ability to do the things you want to do. All the roles you play—parent, partner, breadwinner, friend, neighbor, employee, artist, gardener, or volunteer—may have been affected. You may feel that you are on the sidelines of life or that life is passing you by.

You may also feel you are a burden on others when you can't do what you used to do or have to ask for help. You always wanted a meaningful and purposeful life. Now, in your darkest moments, you may wonder whether you want a life at all. On better days, you ask yourself, "How can I get rid of the pain so that I can get on with my life?" But you feel stuck. You may believe that you have tried everything. You may have actually tried everything health care providers have suggested. So, you think to yourself, "I have done what the doctors and other specialists have told me. Why am I still in such pain?"

Or you may have gotten contradictory advice and don't know what advice to heed. One health care professional may have suggested, "You should take things more easily; you are doing too much." Another, however, suggests, "You should keep moving; you aren't doing enough." And then there are well-meaning friends and family. Your significant other may have told you, "You should persevere; you shouldn't allow yourself to be controlled by the pain." Then, a friend tells you, "You should listen to your body." Not much later, your son calls from across the country and tells you,

"Don't go by how you feel; push through it." Whose advice are you supposed to follow?

If the advice of others has stymied you, and you are not sure what to do, you are not alone. What you really need to do is experiment with your body and become your own expert on what and how much activity helps. In this lesson, you will learn to differentiate between the sense and nonsense others may have suggested.

Here we describe the first of many "active coping" strategies that we teach throughout the book, positive strategies that you can use to help manage your pain, such as pacing your periods of activity, balancing rest and activity, keeping track of your progress, and spending time on things you enjoy. Active coping includes things like problem solving, collecting data to inform your actions, managing your emotions, and focusing on your goals. Where you may have relied on "passive coping" in the past—maybe you avoided talking about your chronic pain with others, or you tried to numb your pain with medication and alcohol, avoiding all activities that you feel might increase your pain—now you'll be managing it more actively. You won't necessarily ignore how your body is feeling in the moment, but you'll also be balancing this with daily decision making based on your goals and the positive things you can do.

Knowing what to do about chronic pain is difficult because of its confusing nature, as we described in Lesson 1. Chronic pain can be musculoskeletal, affecting the bones, muscles, ligaments, and tendons. Or it can be neuropathic—that is, affecting either your central or peripheral nervous system (as is common with cancer treatments, shingles [postherpetic neuralgia], spinal nerve compression, poststroke, and painful diabetic neuropathy). Pain can also be present from internal body organs (for example, endometriosis [pelvic], irritable bowel syndrome [gastrointestinal system], angina [cardiac]). Your pain may be one of these or a combination, or its origin may be a complete mystery. If you have gone to a yoga class or stretching class for "normal" people, the teacher may wisely tell the class, "If you feel pain when you do any of the poses, stop." However, with chronic pain, pain cannot be your only guide with regard to most activities.

Chronic pain may always be present, but you may have also noticed that it varies in intensity or comes and goes unpredictably. In this lesson, we will help you learn to deal with this variability and find out what level and type of activity will be best for you. You will also learn about the importance of pacing and that despite any temporary discomfort, you can become active in ways that increase your energy and improve your conditioning and eventually allow you to do what you have to and want to do.

As you progress, it will become clearer to you how you can regain a level of daily functioning you thought you'd never reach. You may even become more able to do some things you were able to do before your pain began—things you may not have even given much thought to at the time; you just did them.

You will learn not only what you can do but also how you can do it better, longer, more efficiently, and without harming yourself or increasing your pain excessively. Yes, we are talking in part about physical exercise, but don't skip to the next lesson or close the book or throw it in the trash. If the word *exercise* has always turned you off and even scares you, think of it as movement and activity. As the saying goes, move it or lose it!

MOVE IT OR LOSE IT!

How long have you experienced pain? Months, years, decades? Have you tried to prevent pain or at least decrease it by doing less? Do you think, If it hurts, don't do it? When you try to prevent or decrease pain by doing less, you may temporarily reduce or prevent it. However, there may be a cost. By moving less, you actually reduce your strength and flexibility. This is because lack of movement immobilizes your muscles, weakens them, and over time, increases disability. Over a few months of decreased movement, more activities will become difficult and will begin to cause pain. More things will cause or increase your pain. This additional pain is likely not related to the original cause of pain but to weakened muscles (see Figure 2.1).

This may not make sense to you now. After all, you have learned through experience that certain movements will increase your pain. So, you stopped doing them. This appears to be a rational strategy. You know that rest is a necessary condition for healing and recovery. So, you rest. Again, this appears to be a rational strategy.

In one sense, it is. In cases of acute pain following an obvious injury, a brief period of rest (several days at most) in the form of inactivity may be useful. But even in these cases, inactivity for more than a week will lead to weakened muscles and increased disability. Acute and chronic pain are not the same and require different responses from you.

As noted in Figure 2.1, pain leads to reduced mobility, which leads to reduced fitness. For example, have you ever had a broken arm or leg, or do you know someone who has? If you have, you know that after resetting the bone, a cast is usually placed on the limb to keep it from moving in ways that will increase the injury. This lets the broken bone heal. However, this necessary treatment not only keeps the bone from moving, but it also keeps related muscles immobile. When the cast is removed, usually in about 6 weeks, the limb has changed. Comparing that arm or leg with the other that was not injured is clear proof that inactivity causes muscle loss, and muscle loss can increase pain. Another good example of "use it or lose it" involves astronauts:

FIGURE 2.1. Immobility–Pain Cycle

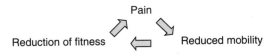

The lack of gravity in space prevents the use of muscles, so when they come back, they have to be carried away on stretchers. It takes time and active rehabilitation for their muscles to recover.

Studies have shown that we lose up to 20% of muscle mass, and hence strength, each week that we fail to make use of our muscles (Kortebein, Ferrando, Lombeida, Wolfe, & Evans, 2007). And if you do not use your muscles, there will be a reduction not only in muscle strength but also in flexibility and endurance.

You may be leery of where we seem to be headed. Instead of resting, you may have done the opposite at times—pushed yourself hard, following the command to "just do it!" But then you have felt much worse for days afterward. Try to suspend judgment for a time, however, when it comes to this lesson. Try to trust that we're not headed in that direction at all.

Being open-minded, you are considering that maybe rest is not always best for healing, and at times, it can make things even worse. Perhaps then you will also consider that unpaced activity (namely, activity that does not build up gradually over time), doing too much too quickly and without appropriate preparation, can cause increased injury and disability. So, what are you to do?

BALANCE AND MIND-SET

The answer is "balance"—that golden middle that most of us swing through when we go from one extreme to another. When the balance between what you can do and what you actually do is disturbed too often, your body protests, rightfully. The more this signal is ignored, the more urgent and louder the protest becomes.

Balance is very personal. What is balanced activity for one person is overwork or underwork for another. So, we have to help you find your personal balance: the amount of movement that may have caused some increased discomfort but temporarily decreases pain and improves your ability to function better—that is, engage in more activities—and with less pain in the long run.

We are not saying that this increase in activities won't cause some discomfort, especially at first, but pain will decrease with practice. When you have chronic pain, it may be difficult to differentiate discomfort from pain, but gradually you will learn how to tell the difference.

The action part of this lesson begins by asking you to change the way you approach your pain. Are you willing to change your relationship with your body from enemy to ally?

To achieve this, you may have to change from always doing it yourself to asking others to help. You may have to change your style from rigid to flexible. We are not saying it will always be easy. However, admitting something is difficult can actually be helpful. For example, telling yourself "this should be easy" when it is hard can make things seem even more difficult, and you can get discouraged if the initial efforts don't go as well as you expected. If doing what we advise is hard, let yourself know that it is hard, but persevere.

All real change is difficult, especially change that requires persistence over time, and it may cause discomfort and make you worry about harming yourself. Many people can lose weight, for example, but the difficulty comes in maintaining that loss. The same is true with changes in activity levels. In the first week, your increase in your level of activity may seem "not so bad." But, after the novelty wears off, the difficulty may be felt acutely. It's okay to admit this. The key is to persevere despite discomfort and setbacks.

What about the week you have a fight with your significant other or the day your car doesn't start? Change is hard enough when things are going well, but it becomes even more difficult when things go wrong. Perhaps in these situations, you can give yourself some slack for a day or so, but no more than that. Again, the key is to persevere.

MOVE SMARTER, NOT HARDER

One thing has likely become clear to you over time: If you could have gotten better by doing your best, you would have *been* better a long time ago. This is true even when you have persisted because when something does not work, the natural tendency is to give up or try harder.

In this lesson, we ask you to list the movement-oriented activities you have done and ask yourself, "Why didn't it work?" For example, "Could I have tried too hard? Could I have not tried hard enough? Did I not understand or have all the information I needed to do what I had to do?" Even simple movements or exercises have a learning curve. "Did a life event or stressor interfere with my plan?" This self-knowledge is important because it will help you to be flexible and allow yourself to alter your plan or approach.

In this lesson, we follow Marianne, one of our patients, who had chronic bursitis in her hips, along with other joint problems. Before Marianne worked with us, she felt discouraged. All the remedies suggested by her family doctor failed to bring much relief. She went to a physical therapist for a few sessions, but the exercises felt boring, and Marianne failed to do them regularly. The therapist finally advised that Marianne get involved in water exercise or walking. After that session, Marianne stopped seeing the physical therapist. But she did decide to try her suggestions.

Water sounded more interesting than walking, but Marianne didn't want to have to get up and get dressed, go to the nearest indoor pool, get wet, and then leave in the cold. A walk sounded really boring. After all, what could walking really do?

Over the December holidays, her 80-year-old father-in-law, Don, visited their home. Marianne and her husband had given him the trip as a holiday present because Don had never been to their new home.

Although he was 20 years older than Marianne, Don walked 2 miles in 30 minutes every single day. He was not a braggart, and before his visit, Marianne never knew he had a walking regimen. In the winter and the heat of the summer, he mall-walked, but in good weather, he preferred being outdoors. In Marianne's area, they were having a mild winter, so Don walked outside during his visit.

Marianne was impressed. If he could do it, she thought, being so much older than she, she could do it too. After Don left, she bought a good pair of running shoes (running shoes are suggested for walkers because of the cushioning they provide). Then she marked out a 2-mile path around their neighborhood. She set her goal (Don's regimen), looked at her watch, and walked the 2 miles in just over 45 minutes. She felt great. The next morning, however, she woke up with tremendous pain in her hips and stayed in bed for 3 days afterward. She felt completely hopeless.

Marianne took only age into account. Because the physical therapist, whom she no longer saw, had once suggested walking, she didn't think it could do any harm. Much later, after consulting us at our pain clinic, she realized she had tried to do too much too soon. But Marianne's journey didn't stop before she saw us. She kept the water workout in the back of her mind. (To be continued.)

ACTIVITY—HOW TO LOVE IT AGAIN

The first step in making activity or movement enjoyable is a mental step. You will have to work on changing the way you view activity by thinking of it as a "want" or "choice" rather than a "must" or "should." You may not think that such wording makes a difference. But listen to how it feels when you say to yourself, "I get to do this" rather than "I must do this." Try talking to yourself (thinking) this way for a week and see what a difference it makes in your attitude, not just about activity but about your life in general. Choosing to do something rather than pressuring yourself to do it will reduce stress—and in turn, decreased stress will decrease your awareness of pain. We discuss stress more in Lesson 3, and we return to a discussion about the impact of our thoughts in Lesson 7.

Second, you'll benefit by changing the way you view "good days" and "bad days," both of which people with chronic pain frequently have. Why do we suggest this? If you have had good days and bad days, you may have found that on the good days you try to catch up on what you feel you have neglected on the bad days. So, you push yourself on the good days only to find that you are exhausted and unable to do much of anything on the next day. Over time, this pattern of pushing yourself on good days and then being too exhausted to do much of anything on the following days will make your pain worse. Remember Marianne's walking routine and her experience. You will also find that you have fewer good days and more bad ones if you continue in this way.

Instead of viewing days as good or bad, think of them as "easy days" or "challenging days." When you feel better, it doesn't mean you *are* better, and when you feel bad, it doesn't mean you *are* bad. On both kinds of days, try to keep to a regular schedule of activity. If problems continue, you might want to cut back on the amount of exercise, but don't view this as an excuse for giving up. Get back on your planned exercise schedule as quickly as possible and try to stick with it. We have more to say about this later in this lesson. But for now, let us reassure you: We know you can't do the same thing on easy days as on challenging days. Later, we describe how on challenging days, you will still stay active, though you might have shorter periods of exertion followed by longer periods of rest and recuperation.

The challenge is to pace yourself, maintaining a reasonable, consistent schedule of activity. Sure, you may do somewhat less on both the easy days and the challenging days at first, but by pacing yourself, you will be able to accomplish more than you did when you pushed yourself too hard on one day and then were laid up afterward. More important, by not overexerting yourself on the easy days, you will be able to have a greater number of days when you feel better (note that we did not say totally pain free).

GETTING STRONGER

What you do often and at a low level (a short amount of time or short distance) will make you stronger; what you do rarely and for too long makes you weaker. If you walk often and briefly on your bare feet, you will get calluses, but if you walk too long on your bare feet, you will get blisters. So, no matter what you feel, whether it is a bad or a good day, try to achieve a balance, and do not let your activity level on easy and challenging days differ too much from each other.

In Figure 2.2, we have illustrated the process of exertion and recovery. When you begin, your exertion will be of short duration, followed by periods for recovery. Over time, the periods of exertion (activity) will increase, whereas the time required for recovery will be reduced.

FIGURE 2.2. Exertion and Recovery: More and More Exertion and Less Recovery Time

When you start pacing yourself, your blocks of time for exertion and recovery look like this:

Exertion	Recovery	Exertion	Recovery	Exertion	Recovery	Exertion

After a few weeks, your recovery time may be shorter:

Exertion	Recover	Exertion	Recover	Exertion	Recover	Exertion

After a few months, your recovery time may shorten even more:

Exertion	Rec	Exertion	Rec	Exertion	Rec	Exertion

After another few months, it is possible you may be able to have fewer recovery periods and longer lasting periods of exertion:

Exertion	Recovery	Exertion	Recovery	Exertion

Many people set a kitchen timer or pay attention to their watch on their good days so that they won't unintentionally overdo it. People who work at computers all day have used the same trick to remind them to stretch or walk around every 20 minutes or so. Working at a computer without frequent stretching can lead to chronic pain problems (for example, in the shoulders and back) or worsen already existing pain.

In yo-yo dieting, dieting that leads to reduced weight at first but increased weight after going off the diet, regaining weight previously lost is then followed by yet another diet. The process repeats itself, with no sustained reduction in weight, which has been shown to be harmful. Being too active on one day, followed by being too passive on other days is bad for your health as well. The important thing, as described earlier, is to find the right balance between doing too little and too much. Before we tackle the most important tool in achieving balanced pacing, let's return to Marianne to see what *not* to do.

Marianne needed more physical therapy after she overdid the walking. The therapist again suggested gentle water walking. So, Marianne decided to look into water exercise courses available in her community. She finally found a drop-in class geared for participants over age 55, so she thought this would work.

The first class she attended on Monday was great. The teacher had arranged for the water to be warm, and Marianne found that getting dressed and going out didn't feel so bad. That night, she slept soundly for the first time in months. She was tired because she had exercised and because she had changed her usual routine by getting out at an appointed time and being with other people.

The second class was on Wednesday. This time, Marianne was familiar with the moves, so she could focus more on working as hard as the others in the class. She couldn't keep pace with them yet, but she tried to do her best. She assumed she would be at their level soon.

Marianne rested until the next class on Monday. This time, she was determined to keep up with the class. After all, water would cushion her joints (or so a magazine article said), and she reminded herself that there were people much older than she in the class.

The following day she felt as bad physically as she had felt after her first 45-minute walk. Emotionally, she felt even worse. Marianne felt she had "failed" again and wanted to give up, telling herself, "What's the use? I made myself worse by exercising."

Marianne forgot that, as with the walking, age is not the only factor to consider when signing up for a class. Is the class geared to beginners? That is an important consideration. Is the teacher credentialed? Has he or she worked with individuals with injuries or chronic pain?

Marianne's group consisted of people at all levels of conditioning. Marianne's teacher had worked with seniors and was good at communicating with them and picking appropriate activities. She also had excellent water aerobics training in terms of safety and movements for each muscle group, but she had no experience with rehabilitative water work.

Marianne was unaware that as we grow older, particularly when we have chronic pain or injuries, the time between strenuous classes may have to be scheduled differently. Monday and Thursday, rather than Monday and Wednesday, would have been better for Marianne. Finally, Marianne didn't realize that a class can bring out the need to keep pace with others, even if one is not competitive. So, let's carefully examine now what Marianne would later learn—the steps involved in pacing.

HOW TO PACE YOURSELF

The initial step in pacing is to select an activity that you would like to do or that you would like to do more. The second is to develop a baseline—that is, define where you are now with regard to that activity. The third step is to set short-term goals and assess progress. And the fourth is to set longer term goals and continue the assessment process. Let's see how each of these steps breaks down.

Pick One Activity

Begin with just one activity (you can add more later). This can be a chore, or it can be a hobby or a form of exercise. Perhaps you would like to do more housework or gardening than you are currently doing. For some people, an orderly house and a neat garden is a real stress-reducer. Perhaps you would like to do volunteer work in a community agency, senior center, or school. If you have children at home, perhaps you would like to be more involved in their activities.

Selecting the right first activity is important. It should be something that is realistic and something you really want to do as well. If you choose something too hard, you will feel discouraged. If you choose something distasteful (for example, doing more cooking when you didn't like to cook even before your pain problem began), you will not have an experience that you will look forward to. Later on, you can take on tasks that don't appeal to you but need doing nonetheless. But first, choose something realistic and desirable.

It doesn't have to be a big or dramatic activity or project. Perhaps you have been bedbound. An increase in activity may simply be getting up and walking around the bed one time. Perhaps you only move from one chair to the sofa, then to a chair at the table, and to bed. An increase in activity would be walking around the room several times. Someone with serious back problems should not carry heavy weights, but making the bed may be an achievable goal. Someone with shoulder tendon problems should not lift large numbers of plates at a time onto a high cabinet shelf, but unloading the dishes one by one from the dishwasher for 5 or 10 minutes and then stacking them on the counter can help.

You may be thinking that what we have been describing accomplishes too little: "How am I ever going to accomplish anything at this pace?" Please don't think that these small activities will not eventually lead to something greater. Trust us—they will. What you are doing, in the beginning, is getting a taste for success and gradually building stamina.

If you are more active currently, you may want to consider more demanding exercises. If you have not exercised for a long time, a few forms of exercise will likely be appealing. Our advice is to choose the one that is simplest and that you dislike the least. The following are a few forms of exercise that our patients have found the least objectionable when they first started exercising:

- walking on a treadmill or other flat surface while listening to music, a podcast, or an audiobook;

- swimming at a leisurely pace;

- doing gentle stretching exercises;

- working with small handheld weights (for example, 1–2 pounds);

- simply walking in water at an indoor pool; or

- doing gentle yoga or one-on-one Pilates exercises (be sure to ask the qualifications of the instructor because exercises such as yoga and Pilates can cause injury if not done correctly and under adequate supervision).

If you tend to be competitive, it is best to stay away from any group activities for a while. Chances are higher that you will not overextend yourself when you have set reasonable goals than if you try to keep up or compete (even unknowingly) with others.

However, if you have an activity "buddy" with the same level of endurance and speed, it can make some activities more pleasurable. You can also encourage each other on days when you don't feel like moving. But if someone else's endurance or speed is above your level, you can fall into the same trap of trying to keep up with a friend as you would in a group activity.

Think about the exercises we have discussed. Keep in mind that almost any form of movement that is not specifically contraindicated by your health care provider will be helpful if you do it gradually. However, whereas exercise is one of the best ways to build stamina, it is not necessary to choose exercise in the beginning. It is most important to choose an activity that you can and will do and that you find appealing and motivating.

Develop Your Baseline

The second step in pacing is deciding on a reasonable amount of time to spend during your first week of increased activity or on how much exercise you will try to do (for example, distance walked, number of repetitions). To do this, you must first develop your baseline.

A *baseline* is simply what you are able to do now in your selected activity. This baseline is the activity level that you will gradually build on. Most people have no idea of what they can normally do. But determining this baseline is critical for you to progress.

To illustrate how developing a baseline works, let's look at weight management programs for a moment. When people start a well-designed program, they are often counseled to write down what they normally eat for a week. They are told not to change it, just to record it.

You are going to do the same with your chosen activity, but not for a week, just for 2 days. If you have already been doing some of the activity you have chosen, simply do what you normally do and stop when you normally stop. Write down how you feel physically and emotionally before and after the activity. If it is an activity you do daily, we suggest you record the activity on both an easy day and on a difficult day. Other than this, please do not do anything different with regard to this activity than you would normally do.

For example, if your chosen activity is walking, establish your baseline by starting from a fixed starting point. Go for a walk as far as you can go, taking into account that you also have to go back. It is better to go twice for a shorter distance than once too long and too far. Count your steps and time yourself. Walk as energetically and buoyantly as possible and make sure you have adopted a good posture with equally divided weight. There are many available applications (apps) you can download on your cell phone that can give you feedback on all kinds of activities, including walking, cycling, running, and swimming. These can help you track your time and distance and show your progress over time—some even include music or game-like features to keep you engaged.

If you are beginning a new activity, plan to do 10% to 20% less than you estimate you can do without a significant increase in the amount of pain or fatigue you are now experiencing. For example, if you decide to go for a walk and you think you can walk for 5 minutes, walk only 4. This will help you not overexert yourself in the desire to get started. Do this on both an easy day and a difficult day. Record in your journal or notebook how you felt before and after, physically and emotionally, on both days.

At first, you may only be able to move for a few minutes or do a few repetitions of an exercise (for example, gently stretching your neck from side to side five times, performing three sit-ups, walking a quarter of a block). This is absolutely fine. The important thing is to have a plan that you have started!

Set Weekly Goals

The next step is to set a goal for the activity or exercise for each day of the first week you plan to begin increasing your activity level. Try not to put this off too long. However, don't start a new activity program during a week that is packed with obligations already (for example, holidays or family birthdays). We want you to experience some success!

For the first 2 or 3 days, we suggest you set your goals at your baseline level. This will allow you to monitor (keep track of) how you are doing on consecutive days. We expect you will feel *some* discomfort, so don't be alarmed. For most people, this discomfort is caused by using muscles that have weakened over time by lack of or reduced use. By reasonably increasing your activity level, you are not doing yourself any harm! Don't get discouraged—over time you will feel less and less discomfort even as you increase your activities.

As recommended earlier, whether you are having a good day or a bad day, try to stick to your initial plan as much as possible. Let your goal of recovery be your guide, not your initial level of discomfort after increasing your activity level.

However, we should emphasize that discomfort and serious increases in pain are not the same thing. Gauge your discomfort each day. If it is minor to moderate, don't worry. If it is significant or if you must rest for a long time before you recover from the activity, you are likely doing too much and have to cut back. If an activity gives some discomfort but the recovery becomes shorter and shorter, that's what counts. It means you are building stamina.

An important part of beginning to increase your activity level is paying close attention to the amount of rest you need between activities. Your weekly schedule of activities (which includes your daily schedule) should be a balance of more active and less active days. Your body will rest and refresh during the less active days. It will build strength and endurance on the more active days. The key is to not under- or overstress your capacity. This is true for activities in a single day as well.

Let's say you are trying to increase the number of household chores you are doing. You will have to build in adequate rest time if you plan to do two chores. For example, vacuuming for 15 minutes once in the morning, followed by a half-hour break, followed by 15 minutes of unloading the dishwasher may be reasonable for you. But doing both back to back, for a total of 30 minutes' activity at a stretch, may cause too much of a strain in the beginning. Eventually, you will build up to 30 minutes of housework in one stretch. But it is particularly important not to overdo it in the beginning.

It is also important to keep in mind which basic muscle groups you are working when you are doing more than one activity in a day. Say, for example, you have decided to exercise using light weights. People who lift heavier weights to keep fit are told not to work the same muscle groups 2 days in a row. Typically, they allow 24 hours before working those muscles again (as they get older, they may need 36–48 hours of recovery time).

This is true for light weights as well. Your muscles should feel a little achy the day after you have worked them; this is normal and a sign that they are becoming stronger. Even if you don't feel achy, you should allow at least 24 hours of recovery time before working these muscles again. If you want to do something the next day, do something that works a different set of muscles. For example, if you lift one-pound hand weights one day, perhaps you can walk a block or so (depending on your baseline) on the next day. This allows you to strengthen both your upper-body and lower-body muscles.

However, you shouldn't allow too much rest time between periods or days of being active. Even professional athletes must watch out for this. For example, elite cyclists vary the intensity and type of activities they engage in. When there is a rest day in the Tour de France bicycle race, the racers continue to exercise, although they might not ride their bikes at all on that day. If the cyclists did not stay active and spent their entire day in bed, the next day, their legs would feel like lead, they would ache, and their performance would suffer.

The key for you is to find that ideal balance between resting too much and resting too little, doing too much and doing too little. What used to be acceptable when you did not have chronic pain (for example, ignoring the pain, and pushing ahead without rest) will have a negative effect when the pain is chronic. The more you do this, the less you will achieve. The same goes for excessive rest. Too much rest leads to muscle weakening and less strength, endurance, and flexibility. The result is that more things become difficult, leading to more inactivity—a vicious circle.

Finally, keep in mind that it is important to increase activities that involve areas of your body where you are not experiencing any pain. Ask yourself, "What parts of my body and what movements cause me the least pain?" When you exercise these areas, it has a positive influence on the rest of your body, including the parts where you most experience pain. Such activities stimulate breathing and the circulation of blood throughout the body. Afterward, you are better able to relax, and this relaxation enables more energy for the things you enjoy, as we discuss in Lesson 3. In short, one part of a reasonable exercise program is to make strong body parts stronger. Indirectly, this will benefit the weaker and painful parts of your body.

Set Monthly Goals

After the first week, set goals so that you are slowly increasing the amount of time you are doing an activity or increasing the number of times you do it. If you are having problems meeting your initial goals—for example, if you have excessive pain or fatigue—cut back and work more slowly. But keep moving ahead.

No two people are the same or change at the same rate, and this makes it particularly important to develop an activity plan that is suited to you personally. You can consult with your doctor or physical therapist if you need more help in developing realistic goals. But remember that only you know whether you tend to go at things too hard and then burn out or whether you're too easy on yourself and are therefore unlikely to achieve much, even over an extended period.

If after increasing an activity (such as a chore or a hobby), you decide to add an exercise program, remember to get a baseline, start slowly, and build gradually. If you don't take a daily walk now, don't try to cover six blocks your first time out.

Again, if you are the kind of person who tends to go to extremes, be careful not to overdo it, no matter which activities you chose. Don't be afraid of a little discomfort, but don't be reckless either!

If you are progressing slowly and are still in a lot of pain after exertion, decrease your levels of activity below your initial baseline. Do not immediately conclude, "That is absolutely worthless. I am already doing so little." Remember, we are only on Lesson 2, so don't get discouraged. Like any skill, it takes time to reach the goals we set. The more impatient you are feeling, the slower you should go in the beginning. Later on, you can push yourself a little harder. But for now, trust our advice.

A note about the timing and location of exercise: If you plan outdoor activities as part of your goal, remember the weather can affect your eagerness to follow the plan. What may seem reasonable in the warm early summer may be less so in a cold, snowy winter. What seems great on a sunny day may look less desirable when there are heavy rain showers. So, try to have back-up plans to accommodate different weather conditions. The weather should not be an excuse for backing off from your plan of activities. Remember Marianne's father—he had a plan for walking that he stuck to summer and winter. In the summer, he walked outside, and in the winter, he walked in a mall.

Gradually Increase Activity

Once you have some experience with increasing activity levels without undue pain, you can try increasing them at a brisker pace—for example, increasing the activity 10% to 20% or by 2- to 3-minute increments on a biweekly or weekly basis. However, do not increase at this level if you are doing light weight lifting. Weight lifting requires slower increases in time or intensity.

In general, remember that the human body is not built to handle extreme changes. For example, if you've ever traveled across the country or overseas, you can tell how difficult it is for your body to adjust to the sudden time change. You might also think of someone who is active during the warmer months but who becomes a couch potato during the winter. When the first nice day of spring arrives, he spends the day playing golf. The sun feels so good and the movement so natural, he forgets he is using muscles that haven't been worked for several months. Each year it comes as a surprise when he feels stiff and achy the following day. Later in the season, he may not feel the same way because the muscles involved in golfing have been strengthened. The same is often true for avid gardeners. The first week of glorious spring can cause a week of agony for knees and hips. And these are people who do not have chronic pain!

Once you have mastered progressing slowly and with consistency, you may be able to increase your activity level gradually every other day. But monitor yourself for signs of overfatigue and pain.

Track Your Progress Over Time

If you have kept daily records of activities and rest periods, you may find it encouraging to see visually how you are progressing over time. Some people find it helpful to keep track of progress using a chart. At the end of this lesson, we offer a blank activity chart you can copy and fill in with the number of minutes you performed your activity or distance traveled (for example, walking or swimming). If you want to see your progress over time, you can create a spreadsheet to record data from several weeks' worth of activity charts and make a bar or line graph from your data. Many fitness apps will do this for you automatically, using data you enter manually or data collected from wearable devices.

A FEW CAUTIONS

To recap the most important points in pacing: When increasing activity levels, develop a baseline and build up slowly and with respect for your body. Once you have set your daily and weekly goals, you should try to stick to them, if possible. Do not do more of your activity (even on easy days), and do not do less, unless you are having a particularly challenging day. In those cases, decrease by 10% to 20% (or more, if necessary), but try not to completely stop being active that day. You should stay in the optimal level of activity, which means neither overdoing nor underdoing what you are capable of. On that note, let's see how Marianne's journey ended.

When Marianne consulted us, we explained that her problems with activity were not due to increasing her activity levels but doing so in an unbalanced way. We agreed with her physical therapist's initial recommendation for walking, but we worked with her to develop a baseline first. We asked her what she thought was a reasonable time or distance she could walk slowly. She thought for a while and then said 15 minutes. Because we could tell she tended to overestimate her readiness, we advised her to try only 10 minutes the first week in establishing her baseline and to monitor herself carefully for an exacerbation of pain. She then asked about two 10-minute walks a day. Again, we told her to start with only one 10-minute walk a day.

Then she asked about adding water aerobics. Couldn't she walk in the morning and do some water exercises in a class in the afternoon? Because she, like many other people, have a hard time not overdoing it in a group situation, we suggested avoiding those classes until she had more experience getting to know her capabilities and limitations. We also did not want her to experience failure in trying NOT to keep up with others at this point. In short, we wanted her to experience success this time! And you will be happy to know that she did.

The Negative Effects of Others' Responses

Perhaps people close to you (including family and friends) were concerned at first when you tried to increase your activity level and became less than supportive when they did not see the improvements they expected. They may even have begun to exert pressure on you, which is not helpful. They may be well-meaning, but if they do not have chronic pain themselves, they cannot know what you are experiencing, and they don't know that you typically put yourself under enough pressure as it is.

For the time being, it is best to start your new level of activity in a quiet way. Don't tell anyone apt to have too high expectations that you are beginning a new program. It is more important in the beginning that you learn to enjoy movement once again than for you to chance a nonsupportive "support network." Of course, before you start exercising to any extent, you should discuss details of your exercise program with your physician or physical therapist. As mentioned at the beginning of this book, our advice is not a substitute for the advice of your health care provider.

You Will Have Setbacks

When you set up an activity or exercise program, you will likely have setbacks at times, when things don't always go as planned (we discuss this again in Lesson 10). It's helpful to know that this is a normal part of the change process. Those on a food plan may follow it rigorously for 3 weeks and then suddenly eat twice their allotted salt intake in one day. Falling off and getting back on the horse almost always accompanies progress at certain points. Even if you do everything perfectly correctly, you will sometimes experience unexpected flare-ups of increased pain. Or you will have 3 highly stressful days in a row (especially around the holidays or family gatherings).

Nothing seems to work well with an all-or-nothing approach. Pushing yourself with "musts" doesn't work as well as encouraging yourself to start your day over, even if it is 3:00 in the afternoon when you do so.

As mentioned in the first part of this lesson, systematic and gradual expansion of activities may initially cause your experience of pain to increase somewhat as you use unused muscles. Ultimately, however, the discomfort and pain will decrease as you improve your strength and endurance. For some, even if the overall decrease in pain seems minor over time, you will notice that more has become possible with less effort. And, the more reasonably active you are, the less you will tend to focus on the pain and the more you will enjoy daily life. The effort and concentration that used to go into protecting yourself might first go into strengthening areas adjacent to the area in which the pain occurs. For example, someone with a weak and painful back has to begin by strengthening the abdominal (stomach), arm, and leg muscles.

SUMMARY

- Pain threatens your ability to function. You may have received a lot of contradictory information about movement and exercise with pain. Therefore, you have to learn how, despite the pain, you can exercise to increase your energy and improve your conditioning.

- Rest is not always best for healing, and at times it may make things even worse. Bodily activity has a beneficial effect.

- Inactivity is only useful in cases of acute pain when there is an obvious injury.

- Exercise may increase discomfort at first because you are using muscles that are weak and out of shape. As you build them up, you should feel less and less pain, *but not immediately*. However, pain is sometimes a signal of overload or an indication that you are doing too much for too long.

- It's easy to do too much if you are feeling good. You can develop movement anxiety due to bad experiences. Then you may end up doing too little when you are feeling bad.

- Don't think in terms of "I must." If you put yourself under too much pressure, every form of physical exercise will ultimately become one you cannot stand.

- Keep a record and maintain a daily schedule and program for you to get ahead. Your possibilities for movement grow when you responsibly seek your limits and build up gradually.

- Discover your general baseline: a daily program with a good balance of activities (exertion) and short periods of rest.

- You might consult a health professional to help you set up your daily program or review one you have created.

- Relapses and setbacks will occur periodically, so allow for a possible relapse or setbacks after some initial success. Plan how you will deal with any setbacks before they occur.

- Don't get discouraged! A failure or a relapse requires encouragement rather than anger and giving up.

QUESTIONS TO CONSIDER

1. What does your normal day look like, and was it different in the past? If so, how?
2. Is there a difference between listening to your body and letting yourself be guided by your feelings? What is the difference?
3. How will you determine your baseline?
4. How can you expand beyond your baseline? What will you do when you cannot increase your activity any further?
5. What will you do if you feel increased pain when you exercise?
6. Which of your body parts and what movements cause you the least pain? In what way can you practice and make the strong parts stronger?
7. Are you tempted to tell yourself, "I must"? Why is *must* so harmful? How will you cultivate a healthy mind-set around activity?

8. Try walking (or other exercises) on your own on some days and with a partner ("buddy") on others. Which did you like best?

HOME ACTIVITIES

1. How many hours a day do you spend sitting, lying down, standing, and exercising, including doing household chores? Record in the following spaces the number of hours you do each of these. Be honest with yourself.

    – Sitting _____ hr
    – Lying down _____ hr
    – Standing _____ hr
    – Exercise or chores _____ hr
    – Total   24 hr

2. Look at your current activity baseline alongside your pain levels at different times of day. Figure 2.3 is an example chart for 8:00 to 11:00 in the morning.

    Figure 2.4 is a blank chart for you to fill in. Record how you spend your time and what activities you are doing at different times. Place a mark in each row indicating your current activities throughout the day and rate the level of pain you currently experience doing those activities (0 = *no pain* to 10 = *most severe pain*). You can download additional blank charts from http://pubs.apa.org/books/supp/turk.

    As you fill in the chart, think about how the time of day and your energy level at different times of day affects your pain. What if you moved an activity you usually do in the morning to the afternoon or vice versa?

3. You can also use the chart in Figure 2.4 to create a plan where you balance activity and rest patterns. You can copy the chart and add and modify the times for activity and rest over days and weeks as you work with this program and beyond. Remember to increase the amount of activity and decrease rest time *gradually*. Don't overdo it, but try for steady progress that best fits you.

FIGURE 2.3. Example Activity Baseline Chart for 8 a.m. to 11 a.m.

Time	Lie	Sit	Stand	Walk	Activity	Pain 0–10
8:00–8:30am	X	X	X	X	Wake up, get up, shower	6
8:30–9:00		X			Breakfast, read paper	4
9:00–9:30			X	X	Clean	8
9:30–10:00			X	X	Shop	7
10:00–10:30			X	X	Arrange the wardrobe	4
10:30–11:00		X			Listen to music	0

FIGURE 2.4. My Current Activity Baseline

DATE: _____   Scale 0–10: 0 = *no pain,* 10 = *most severe pain*

Time	Lie	Sit	Stand	Walk	Activity	Pain 0–10
6:30–7:00 a.m.						
7:00–7:30						
7:30–8:00						
8:00–8:30						
8:30–9:00						
9:00–9:30						
9:30–10:00						
10:00–10:30						
10:30–11:00						
11:00–11:30						
11:30–12:00						
12:00–12:30 p.m.						
12:30–1:00						
1:00–1:30						
1:30–2:00						
2:00–2:30						
2:30–3:00						
3:00–3:30						
3:30–4:00						
4:00–4:30						
4:30–5:00						
5:00–5:30						
5:30–6:00						
6:00–6:30						
6:30–7:00						
7:00–7:30						
7:30–8:00						
8:00–8:30						
8:30–9:00						
9:00–9:30						
9:30–10:00						
10:00–10:30						
10:30–11:00						

4. Create your plan for one activity you will work on. To track your progress, use a chart like the one shown in Figure 2.5. List the activity at the top of the chart, and put the days of the week along the horizontal line. Put the number (distance, time, or repetitions of the task) on the vertical line beginning with your base level (what you can do comfortably or feel reasonably

FIGURE 2.5. My Activity Tracker

Activity: _____

Set the numbers along the left side as needed to start with to your baseline number of minutes or repetitions. For example, if you can currently walk for 10 minutes, start the numbering at 10 and go up. Increase your time, distance, pace, and/or repetitions by increments that are realistic and healthy for you.

	Sun	Mon	Tues	Wed	Thurs	Fri	Sat
15							
14							
13							
12							
11							
10							
9							
8							
7							
6							
5							
4							
3							
2							
1							

Possible problems that will interfere with my activity:

_____
_____
_____

How I will deal with problems that interfere:

_____
_____
_____

comfortable doing now), and for the next week record your progress on the chart. You can photocopy this sample chart and use it for any number of activities or exercises, over multiple weeks. You can also download it from http://pubs.apa.org/books/supp/turk.

- Make sure to list the problems you anticipate will interfere with doing the exercise.
- Describe how you will deal with each of these problems if they do come up.

If you haven't started to exercise, after 2 or 3 weeks of increasing your other activities, begin to incorporate exercise into your weekly routine. Follow the guidelines for pacing detailed in this lesson.

Learning to Relax

The truth is that taking the time to be still and reflective actually increases productivity and gives more joy to what you're doing when it's time to take action again.

—MARIA ERVING

With continual pain, you may feel that you are waging a battle with your body all day, every day. Pain may feel like the enemy—a monster that makes you afraid of tomorrow, keeps you from sleeping tonight, and stops you from enjoying today. A result of this battle is that you may feel all kinds of negative emotions (feelings) that add to your pain.

You want to fight the pain monster or run away from it, but you find that you can't fight, and you can't flee. So, you feel stuck and demoralized.

When you try to relax, it feels like a car in neutral gear with someone else stepping on the gas. Your engine revs up, but you can't move forward no matter how hard you step on the gas. High arousal and tension levels leave you too exhausted to move.

Along with this internal pressure, you may feel pressure from others to be more productive. It may be true that your family, friends, children, health care providers(s), employer, and insurance company are, in fact, making life more difficult by their lack of understanding. Or you may be reading things into others' looks or words, but you are so exhausted, you don't realize this. If you are a breadwinner (sole wage earner) in the family or your own sole support, you may also develop financial problems that add to your distress. If you are the home manager, you may feel guilty that you can no longer do as much or as well as you used to. You worry that you may never get better, and you worry that others are having similar thoughts.

These ongoing stressors and others all interfere with your ability to get adequate rest and a good night's sleep. This, in turn, creates another vicious

49

circle. It is much easier to cope with pain when you are rested, but because you never seem to feel rested anymore, your coping is impaired. This leads to even more problems.

In this lesson, you will learn about these and other causes of tension and restlessness. More important, you will learn the positive effect of relaxation on your energy balance and your experience of pain. Most important, you will learn how to truly relax again—despite your level of pain at the moment.

When you increase your ability to relax and achieve more restful sleep, you will begin to feel more energetic, and you will gain a new sense of control over your life. You will notice that being more relaxed lessens the severity of your pain and decreases the negative effects of pain on your life.

THE ENERGY BALANCE

In today's fast-paced, rapidly changing, and overcommitted world, it is difficult for most people to maintain the balance between effort and relaxation. We are bombarded every day with seemingly endless amounts of information. Cell phones have been a wonderful boon in terms of being able to coordinate schedules, contact help when a car breaks down, or let your employer or family know if you're going to be late. But they have had the unintended effect of making people feel that they must always be available and they must always keep up.

A minority of families can get along with one person staying at home to keep the household running. But most families need two incomes, especially if they have children to clothe, feed, and educate. Single parents are under tremendous stress. The majority of people try to do too much but feel they have no alternative.

When you add chronic pain to this equation, you can see why you may feel stressed and overwhelmed most of the time. To help, well-meaning people tell you that you have to take time for yourself to reduce stress. However, you often find that if you do, you are too exhausted to enjoy it. Shopping is no longer a pleasant pastime but a tedious hunt—for a parking place, for a bargain, and then for a place to put that bargain.

Without meaning to, most of us get caught up in this hectic pace until our bodies become overloaded and, as a consequence, go "on strike." We are unable to sleep, we come down with a cold or the flu, or we wrench a muscle. People who are living with chronic pain are not immune to additional illnesses or injuries.

There is no such thing as a life without tension. But there is an optimal level of stress. Without changes that call for adaptation, life would be boring. But too much stress over too long a period is not good for anyone, especially a person with chronic pain, like you.

When you have chronic pain, you often feel guilty about the idea of relaxing when you are contributing less than you used to. But you are no different in your need to recharge your batteries and leave the stress behind for a while. In the previous lesson, we emphasized the value of activity. In this lesson, we emphasize the other part of the equation—true rest and relaxation.

ARE YOU OVERSTRESSED?

How do you know whether you are indeed overstressed? Here are some clues:

- You want to do many things at the same time,
- you consistently want to do more than you are capable of,
- you give up and want to do nothing at all, and
- you attempt to take control of things that are not under your control (other people, places, and events).

Stress and these symptoms of stress take energy away from you. Think of energy like you think of money. When the expenses are higher than the income, sooner or later, you'll be in financial trouble. When your body uses up more energy than it produces, you will feel physically and emotionally bankrupt.

It may be hard to believe when you think about how you have been doing less and less since your pain began and worrying more and more, but pain itself causes stress. So, living with pain is another stressor, unless you learn how to manage the pain through a balance of activity (described in Lesson 2) *and* relaxation.

If you are having trouble grasping this, think of it this way: When you are overstressed or underrelaxed, the muscles in your body are naturally tense. This means that your body is under too much pressure. This pressure can increase your heart rate and cause shallow breathing, which increases fatigue and leads to feelings of exhaustion. Furthermore, for many people, proper nutrition is the first thing that is sacrificed when they are under stress. They either eat too much, too little, or the wrong foods. In any case, their body is running on the wrong amount or type of fuel. Most important, these effects of being overstressed and under relaxed can increase your pain by affecting what you think, feel, and do, as well as directly affecting your body.

Let's try another example because people are surprisingly resistant to suggestions that they need to relax. When you buy a car, you're interested in whether your car will last over time and whether it has important safety features. You're also interested in whether this complicated machine will need special maintenance. With energy costs skyrocketing, you're most certainly interested in the prospective car's fuel consumption and how this fits in with your budget.

Your body is complex, much more so than your car. If you want your body to have enough fuel to enjoy your life, you have to make it more energy efficient. And you certainly want to conserve fuel so that you can take care of routine activities. This is where relaxation comes in. When your body is tense, your muscles are consuming unnecessary fuel, fuel you need for enjoyment and the requirements of daily life.

CONSERVING ENERGY

The first step in conserving fuel is to learn to know when you are tense and when you are relaxed. This is more difficult than most people think. People are often unaware of their bodies, except for the experience of pain. When you are under tension for extended periods, you are unconsciously tense and unknowingly consuming a great deal of fuel. Tension is both mental and physical. Let's try a small exercise to help you learn how physical tension feels.

Try this. Make a fist with your right hand. Clench your fist tightly. Really squeeze it tight. Feel your fingers pushing into your palm. Hold it there!

Now bring your clenched fist up toward your opposite shoulder and press the fist against your shoulder. Feel the muscles in your right forearm and your biceps (the muscle between your elbow and shoulder) begin to quiver. Hold it there. Count slowly to five: one, two, three, four, five.

This is muscle tension. If you keep this up long enough, it will start to hurt, and you will experience increasing pain, eventually even unbearable pain.

Now, compare how your left hand and arm feel in comparison with your right. Note the different feelings and sensations between the right and the left hands and arms. Your left is in a state of relaxation; your right is in a state of tension, muscle tension.

Now, slowly, relax your fist and arm. Slowly bring your fist down from your shoulder. Let your muscles relax. Move your fingers away from your palm, relaxing your fist. Slowly bring your fist and arm down to rest loosely on the arm of your chair, a table, or your lap.

Do you see how different this feels? This is relaxation. Relaxation feels different to different people. For some doing this exercise, their right hand feels warm. For others, it tingles, feels a bit heavy, or feels very light.

Notice the difference in how your right hand and arm feel now compared with when you tensed them.

Even with this short exercise, you have learned that you have some control over muscular tension—perhaps more than you think—and that you can bring about muscle tension and muscle relaxation through conscious effort to some degree. This means that you have more control over your daily tension levels than you previously thought and that you have power that you have not yet harnessed. In this lesson, we hope to help you learn how to harness your ability to reduce your pain.

SOURCES AND SYMPTOMS OF EXCESS STRESS

Because excess muscular tension is often unrecognized, it is helpful first to learn more about the most frequently occurring sources and symptoms of chronic muscular tension and stress. Be aware that people rarely have all these symptoms and that what is stressful for one person may not be for another.

Next, we list some of the sources of tension people in our practices have shared. As you review these, think of yourself and how they apply to you. Some may be more relevant than others for you, but they are all important to consider.

Sensory Overload

Heavy traffic, noisy groups of people, loud radio and television advertisements, worrying news that bombards you all the time—these make many people tense. Some people with chronic pain report problems with bright lights (especially if they have chronic headaches); others feel greater sensitivity to cold and damp weather (common in people who have pain related to arthritis).

How about you? Stop and think for a moment. Have you noticed a lower tolerance for some forms of sensory stimulation than you had before your pain began? Which ones can you think of that affect you?

Emotional Vulnerability

When people have chronic pain, they commonly feel distressed and overwhelmed, but they often stifle their emotions until they feel they will explode. Then, they may break down and cry or have a fit of temper at unexpected times. These outbursts may be troubling, but it helps to know that they are almost always a result of stored tension.

Some of these negative emotions you feel and may hold in are triggered by the sense of futility you have felt over managing your pain. You may then feel guilty and angry with yourself about mood changes or "irrational feelings" you may experience. Guilt alone is a great stressor.

How has your pain influenced your mood? Do you often feel upset, angry, or depressed? Do you think these feelings affect the intensity of your pain? Some people have difficulty accepting these negative feelings. It is okay to admit these feelings, if only to yourself. You may be thinking it is "easier said than done." But as we discuss later in the lesson and in Lesson 7, you can learn how to become more aware of and how to express and control your feelings more effectively.

You may think you are the only one who has such negative emotions. However, your feelings are not unusual, especially for people with chronic pain. Negative emotions can contribute to increased muscle tension and thereby increased pain. People with chronic pain have often adapted to this by tuning out their body sensations as much as possible.

The first step in dealing with the stress that is depleting your energy is to pay closer attention to your body. By this, we mean that the next time you notice a negative feeling (frustration, anger, worry), begin to pay attention to all your bodily sensations. Do you notice any tension in any of your muscles? Does your body feel numb (except for the pain)? It takes time and practice to tune in to your body in this way, but it is critical to your success in managing your pain.

Once you become aware of the effects of your negative emotions, you can take steps to alter these and ultimately to reduce the intensity of your pain.

When you experience stress, in addition to paying attention to your body, try to catch what you are thinking. Thoughts are fleeting, and it takes practice to catch them. But this skill, too, is critical to practice. We return to the role of thoughts in self-managing your pain in Lesson 7. For now, it is important to simply understand that thoughts and feelings can increase arousal and the accompanying muscular tension and pain and that awareness of bodily sensations and thoughts can help relax muscles and reduce pain.

Uncertainty and Fear

Fears of open spaces, anxiety while traveling in cars and other enclosed vehicles, fear of crossing bridges, fears of going to the dentist, and heightened tension in shopping malls are all quite common in the general population. These fears can be accompanied by a sense of dizziness, shortness of breath, a knot in your stomach, and a rapid heartbeat. This, in turn, can lead to further anxiety and avoidance of situations that cause these distressing sensations. However, avoidance of travel, outings, and social situations can increase feelings of isolation and loneliness and actually increase stress. Avoidance of needed dental care can lead to even greater problems down the line.

Other fears are less specific and can be experienced as "free-floating" anxiety. Common concerns our patients have noted underlying these fears are that (a) their pain will never end, (b) their pain or underlying condition will worsen, (c) they will become progressively more disabled and dependent on others, (d) people won't believe how bad their pain really is, and (e) they're told they will have to learn to live with the pain—but they have been living with it, and they want to live without it or at least be told how to live with it if they must. Have you experienced any such thoughts and fears? If you have, what effect do you think they have on your pain?

Such fears and thoughts often occur spontaneously and are accompanied by rapid, shallow breathing. This type of breathing can occur without awareness and can also increase muscle tension directly and lead to anxiety or feelings of panic. Later in this lesson, we teach you some skills to help you breathe through these stress-provoking situations and feelings so as not to increase your stress, muscle tension, and pain.

Loss of Concentration

Tension, like pain, often interferes with concentration and memory. Some medications for pain can also have these effects. These may be dose dependent (that is, the more medication taken, the worse the side effects you experience), so lowering dosages can sometimes help with cognitive problems. If you think your medication may be causing such effects, you should discuss this with your physician and not change your medication on your own. People with chronic pain often describe their state of mind as being similar to walking around in a fog or being "out of it." Side effects of medication can add to these feelings.

Have you felt a decrease in your ability to concentrate and remember things since your pain began? Do you sometimes feel as if your brain is in a fog? Has your pain affected your memory, your concentration, and your attention span? This is an especially common experience for individuals who have widespread pain affecting multiple areas of the body accompanying a number of other physical and emotional symptoms such as excessive fatigue, bowel problems, and anxiety (for example, fibromyalgia, irritable bowel syndrome, migraine and tension-type headaches, endometriosis, back pain).

Chronic Fatigue

Many people with chronic pain also feel a sense of chronic fatigue or constant tiredness. They start the day feeling tired, so they often wonder, "What's the sense in getting out of bed?" Sitting or standing for a long period may feel daunting, and climbing the stairs seems like climbing a mountain. Every effort seems to be too much to bear. When they push themselves, they feel as if they are engaged in battle, with pressure in their chests and a racing heartbeat.

Much of this is the result of being physically unfit from restricting activity. Using fuel in appropriate ways makes the body more fuel efficient. That is why Lesson 2 was so important, even for chronic fatigue.

Some people try to pep up their overloaded nervous system with stimulants (such as cigarettes, caffeine, or certain prescribed medications). This may help at the moment but leads to more exhaustion later on. It is possible to boost the exhausted body for a short period artificially, but over time, however, these stimulants backfire, overwhelming the nervous system and creating more anxiety and stress. As people become physically dependent and require larger quantities of stimulants to get the same effect, they become more exhausted still. Does any of this sound like you?

Sleep Problems

It seems strange to many of our patients that despite their fatigue, they feel their sleep is not refreshing. Many have trouble falling asleep and staying asleep. Their sleep may be fitful, and they wake up more tired than they were when they went to bed. Some people are not even aware their sleep is disturbed until they ask their partner.

Think about yourself for a moment. How would you describe your pattern of sleep? Do you toss and turn a lot? Do you wake up feeling just as tired as when you went to sleep? We discuss sleep and ways to improve it in detail in Lesson 4.

Stomach and Digestive Problems

Some of our patients report problems with swallowing, feeling "too full," being constipated, having frequent diarrhea, losing their appetite, overeating, or alternating over- with undereating (these symptoms are also hallmarks of a distressing disorder—irritable bowel syndrome—but note that they are also common side effects of many medications used to control pain). They often report an increase in weight, most often because of inactivity and extra snacking to fill up the space pleasurable activities used to occupy. This extra weight makes their bodies less fuel efficient and contributes to tension, fatigue, and lack of energy. It also results in feelings of unattractiveness. For example, one of our patients used to enjoy dancing, but he no longer went dancing because of the increased visible weight he carried. Some turn down routine social invitations that could potentially increase their energy because they are embarrassed about their weight gain. Have you noticed changes in your eating habits and weight since your pain began? We describe some strategies to help with your diet in Lesson 4.

Changes in the Immune System

Some of our chronic pain patients have reported increased problems with infection and allergies, as well as a heightened susceptibility to colds and flu. This typically results from a combination of inactivity, poor diet, and the daily stress of coping with chronic pain, as opposed to the original cause of their pain.

Whereas the immune system must fight germs all the time, the stressors and symptoms described in this section deplete the immune system's arsenal in such a way that the person who experiences chronic pain may be more likely to develop other illnesses.

LEARNING TO RELAX

In short, the inability to relax deeply and regularly is responsible for a range of serious health problems. Relaxation can help replenish this arsenal in addition to helping decrease pain directly. But how exactly does one learn how to relax?

We have already mentioned two major skills involved in learning to relax: bodily awareness of stress and emotions and mental awareness of thoughts that accompany stress. We have much more to say about thoughts in later lessons. In this lesson, we focus on bodily relaxation.

You may be thinking that you have tried to relax but with little effect. Some methods are better than others. Think of whether you have tried any of the following methods.

Alcohol and Other Drugs

Many different classes of drugs are used to treat pain, even though not all drugs that are effective against pain were originally designed for that purpose (see Appendix A for information about medications used to treat pain). Alcohol (yes, alcohol is a drug), antianxiety prescription drugs (for example, valium, clonazepam), and some antidepressant drugs relax the muscles. The result is that feelings of arousal, worry, and tension may be temporarily reduced or suppressed. However, these muscle-relaxing drugs have the disadvantage of physical dependence and tolerance.[1]

If you have been taking such drugs for more than a week, do not stop taking them (perhaps with the exception of alcohol) unless you are under the supervision of a physician. You cannot stop most drugs rapidly or "cold turkey" without your body responding in alarming or harmful ways (e.g., seizures, increased depressive thoughts). As noted, this is not unique to drugs for pain but is true for any medication.

If you start to reduce your drug dosage even under the supervision of a physician, or if you stop drinking alcohol or stop smoking abruptly, you may notice some unpleasant side effects (for example, headache, sweating, flu-like symptoms, difficulty sleeping or concentrating) because of your body's physical dependence. Even stopping caffeine can have strong effects, such as an inability to concentrate and throbbing headaches for over a week. So, if appropriate, it is better to gradually wean yourself from any prescription and nonprescription drugs you are using to reduce stress or pain, with the advice of your physician.

Relaxation Exercises

If you've tried relaxation exercises before and found that they didn't seem to work, ask yourself why they didn't work. It is possible you did not understand when and how to use relaxation exercises or did not practice them long enough to get any benefits. You might have tried them when there was too much going on around you (for example, the television was on, the children were arguing).

There are many ways to relax, and there is no one way that is best for everyone. Some people benefit from relaxation involving imagery (mental pictures), others benefit from video or audio supports or written instructions, and still others need some physical activity while they relax (for example, floating in water, gentle stretching). If you choose a method that is not right for you, you will be unlikely to benefit from it or keep practicing long enough to achieve results.

Learning to relax is a skill; it takes practice. Patients with serious heart problems, for example, are asked to do daily relaxation exercises consistently for 90 days before they can expect to see results. This is because real relaxation

---

[1]Physical dependence occurs when any drug, even blood pressure and thyroid medications, is taken over time. The body adjusts and may require additional amounts to produce the same effect. This is why it is important to gradually decrease the doses of any medications to prevent symptoms such as increased anxiety or sweating from occurring. Tolerance is common. It means that as your body adapts to the drug, you continually need more of the drugs to achieve the same effect. This is true for prescribed drugs as well as alcohol, marijuana, and illicit drugs such as cocaine and methamphetamine.

seems deceptively simple but is actually a skill, like any other, that we have to learn. You must learn what method is right for you—there are lots to try out—to discover which is best for you, and then you must practice, practice, and practice to gain and retain the highest level of benefit.

If you do practice consistently, you may feel out of sorts when you miss a session or feel like you do when you have forgotten to brush your teeth. In the remainder of this lesson, we focus on a few of the many ways to learn to relax. If the ways we describe do not work for you, do not give up. There are a wide variety of audio relaxation tools (some may be available at local libraries, through your smartphone app store, and on the Internet) and also classes in many communities that teach relaxation in different ways, including in groups. In addition, even if you find one that is helpful to you, there may be times when you are disappointed and might want to try one of the other methods we describe here.

There are many different ways to relax your body and your mind. As we noted, there is no one best way to relax. The important thing is to find some means of relaxing that is comfortable for you and use these activities regularly. Relaxing should become just as much a part of your daily routine as getting dressed and brushing your teeth. So, let's get started—remember, you are seeking the best approach(es) for you. Even if you are not sure they will be helpful, try the different ones we describe for a few days to discover what produces the best effects.

Systematic Muscle Relaxation

As you learned earlier in this lesson, some muscles are under your control even if you are not aware of it at the moment. Skeletal muscles fall into this category. There are, however, also muscles that do their work more automatically and without conscious awareness—for example, the internal muscles of the digestive system (stomach and bowels) and your heart muscle, among others. Pay attention to your body right now. Can you feel any tense muscles in your neck, your back, your chest? With practice, you can gain some control over many of your muscles. We provide some detailed exercises to help you relax different muscle groups in Appendix 3.1 at the end of this lesson.

Breathing Correctly

Many people are "chest breathers." That is, they suck in their abdomens and expand their chests with each in-breath. This may be particularly true for women because, in Western cultures, they are taught early in life that "proper" posture is one in which the abdomen is flat at all times.

This posture is difficult to maintain when you are truly relaxing. Diaphragmatic breathing (the diaphragm is just below the ribs), which produces the truly relaxing breath, requires the stomach to move in and out with each breath. If you want to observe natural diaphragmatic breathing, watch infants when they breathe. Their tummies move gently in and out with each breath.

Many people also become shallow chest breathers because of prolonged anxiety, stress, and tension. When tensed, your breathing naturally becomes faster and shallower and comes from the chest. Stress tends to increase tension in the abdominal area, so the diaphragm cannot contract completely, and the abdominal wall cannot move out when taking a breath. Only the chest expands, as a result, causing further tension. How about you? Pay attention to your breathing pattern for a few moments.

The first step in learning to truly relax, the one you need to master before you proceed further, is to practice diaphragmatic breathing. Brief periods of diaphragmatic breathing provide your body's energy needs in two ways. First, this type of breathing is best able to remove the carbon dioxide from your blood. At the same time, it produces oxygen, both great sources of energy. Second, breathing properly ensures the beneficial massage of the abdominal organs. This is why gentle yoga can be effective, as well.

Diaphragmatic breathing can bring about a feeling of calm and relaxation when it is properly practiced. To feel your diaphragm during breathing, place your hand just above your stomach, take a slow deep breath through your nose, and feel the movement of your hand as you do so. As you slowly breathe out through your mouth, you will find yourself relaxing without even trying. Longer and deeper breathing of this sort can make "normal" breathing easier and more relaxed. Put down the book and try this for a few moments. Pay attention to your pattern of breathing. See whether you can increase your diaphragmatic breathing. Notice how this compares with your normal breathing.

When first learning how to breathe in this way, it often helps to lie down on a bed or cushioned floor, knees slightly bent, and place your hands on your stomach. In this way, you can feel the abdomen rise when you breathe in and contract when you breathe out. Try practicing for 10 minutes or so while you are doing something passive in the morning, afternoon, and evening, such as listening to the radio. Appendix 3.2 provides detailed instructions for practice. One man we treated became so good at diaphragmatic breathing that he taught and coached his pregnant wife so she could control her breathing during the delivery of their first child and thus experience less pain.

Along with diaphragmatic breathing, many people find that visualizing images helps them relax. If you want to pair the two relaxation techniques, we have also included a visualization exercise in Appendix 3.3. You can try these out and see how they work for you. In addition to images, some people find focusing on a calming or spiritual word or phrase to be helpful. Remember, there is no best technique for everyone; you are trying to discover what is best for you. You may also find that different methods work better for you at different times.

Keep in mind that becoming more skilled at controlled, relaxed breathing may take some time. So, don't be discouraged if what initially sounds easy is, in fact, a bit difficult. Many of us have a running monologue or dialogue in our heads most of the time, and it takes practice to quiet this voice.

You also may not feel immediate results. The body is not used to this kind of practice. It barely remembers infancy, when this kind of breathing came naturally. With practice, your body will begin to trust your mind again, and some days you will find these exercises both effortless and rewarding.

Attention Diversion

Those who have chronic pain naturally tend to focus on their bodies and their situation too much, on how severe the pain is, and on how much they can or cannot do. This is human nature. We each have the untapped ability, however, to attend to other things and other people, at least some of the time. You can consider some ways to use your intentional focus to distract yourself when your pain is difficult to bear.

If your reaction right now is, "I can't distract myself. My pain is too severe," we gently suggest that you try out some of the exercises and see what happens. You may be surprised. Controlling your attention when you have pain is difficult, and it helps to admit when things are difficult. Also, effective distraction, like controlled breathing, takes time and practice.

There are several ways you can divert your attention. The way diversion works with pain is based on the principle that we cannot focus on everything that is going on around us all the time. For example, while you are reading this lesson, some sounds are likely going on in the background. Stop for a moment and listen. What do you hear? It might be the sound of the fan on your air conditioner or heater. It might be the wind blowing outside your window, traffic noises outside your home, or the ticking of a clock.

In the same way, there are feelings within our body that we fail to pay attention to all the time. For example, you may have a watch on your wrist or ring on your finger. If you do, focus on how they feel against your skin. How about your socks or shoes? How do they feel? How does your back feel against the chair, couch, or bed on which you are reading? You may not notice these sensations until they become the focus of your attention. As they do become the focus, you may not be aware of other sensations on which you were previously focusing.

The important thing about this is to realize that all these sensations and sounds are always going on, but out of habit, we do not pay attention to them; we tune them out. This is because attention can be likened to watching television, listening to the radio, and surfing the Internet. All the stations and websites are there all the time, but we can only tune into and focus on one at a time.

When it comes to our pain, many people do not realize the power of focus and attention, particularly distraction. By distraction, we can choose what will be the focus of our attention for a specific time. You might think that the focus of your attention is your pain. That may be true, but while you are focusing on your pain, you are tuning out everything else going on around you. If you shift to some other things, you may be able to distract yourself from your pain. That does not mean your pain will be gone but that you may be able to reduce the intensity by focusing on other things to capture your attention.

You have probably made use of attention diversion or distraction without even realizing it. You might read books or magazines, study religious materials, listen to music, work on a hobby, play video games, use social media, or listen to someone when they call to talk on the telephone. Sometimes when you do these activities, you may lose track of time or where you are. In each of these cases, your attention is highly focused, and you are likely not aware of many other things going on around you and within you. If this is true for you, know that you are engaging in a habit that has the power to help you manage your pain. There are many free and low-cost forms of distractions, so look into some of the ones available. See whether any interest you and then give them a try. Try to find ones that work best for you. When you do, try to make them a part of your daily routine.

Spiritual Focus: Meditation and Prayer

One way to divert attention from pain and induce a state of relaxation is to focus on some spiritual word, phrase, or prayer or something meaningful to you. When we discussed controlled breathing earlier, we mentioned that spiritual words can be used in conjunction with this type of breathing to help you relax. Prayer by itself or a focus on a religious figure such as Jesus, Mohammed, Buddha, or the spiritual being some call a *higher power* can be tremendously calming. Others find focusing on a sense of oneness with nature to be helpful. In any of these pathways, there are options for meeting with a community of like-minded others or finding an individual practice that gives structure to the experience. If this kind of focus appeals to you, you can focus on whatever you find most meaningful and relaxing.

Sensory Focus

We also tell our patients that if their pain, worries, or seemingly insoluble problems have kept them upset for a long time, it is not possible to let these difficulties go all at once. We ask them to practice visualizing one pleasant experience for a brief period. They are instructed to reach into their memories and recall a happy or peaceful time. They close their eyes and focus on each visual aspect of that scene. We then ask them to focus on the sounds and smells associated with that scene, as well as the tactile memories—what the sun felt like if it was a summer scene, what the cold felt like if it was winter. Try this now, at least once, for a few minutes.

It can also be helpful to see yourself in pleasant places, whether or not you have actually traveled there:

- Picture yourself in the cool of dusk, sitting at the edge of a lake. Look at how the water reflects the light from the moon, feel the cool breeze against your skin, and hear the birds off in the distance.

- Picture yourself walking through a park on a beautiful autumn day. Hear the breeze rustling through the tall trees. Feel your feet sinking into the soft ground as the golden red, yellow, and orange leaves rustle beneath you.

- Picture yourself lying on an uncrowded beach at the ocean. Feel the sun on your face. Hear the breaking of the waves. See the horizon line as you look in the distance. Enjoy the feeling of space around you. Sit up and watch the different tints of blue, green, and gray in the sea. Enjoy the clear blue sky. Perhaps have a cold drink or a Popsicle. Taste it. Savor each drop. Which drink or flavor did you choose?

We are sure you can think of many other scenes once you get the idea. Such relaxing images have a direct effect on muscle tension. Focusing on these can take your mind off your pain, even if for only a brief period. Perhaps you are thinking that, given your pain, you can't do this. Hold back on that thought for a few moments and see what we suggest later.

The particular image you use in coping with pain is *not* the most important thing. The most important thing is to be *involved* in the image so that all your attention is focused on the image and the sensations. Whenever possible, make use of all your senses—vision, hearing, touch, taste, and smell.

As in the breathing exercises, your attention may wander from time to time, and you may occasionally find yourself dwelling on unpleasant sensations or thoughts. But you can gently bring your attention back to the pleasant image or scene when you notice that your attention has wandered.

As you first start this practice or when you practice on challenging days, you may still be somewhat aware of the discomfort or pain. But these will gradually fade into the background as you focus on the sensations associated with the scene. The pain may not totally disappear, but it may be more like the ticking of a clock or the sound of a fan—noticeable but not as irritating.

What would be a pleasant scene for you? What would you include? Pleasant images bring with them a feeling of safety. In Appendix 3.3, we have included a detailed sample of a scene that many people find pleasant. You might read this over and then try to experience it yourself. Once again, you may wish to make a voice recording of yourself reading this scene. Perhaps someone you are comfortable with may be willing to read the scene and record it for you.

If you have trouble coming up with a scene in your mind, look at pictures in nature, outdoors, or travel magazines. Many libraries have such magazines available. Even if you don't use the scene in a focused exercise, just looking at such pictures can be relaxing. The same is true of watching nature shows on television, and they can be "streamed" on many electronic devices.

Keep in mind when you use such scenes that there is no reason for you to feel locked into any one image. If you find the scene you are using to be ineffective or even distressing, you can easily turn it off and switch to another scene. Some images may inadvertently unconsciously recall distressing times in your life that you may have forgotten. Also, some images fade and become less vivid after a while.

You can elaborate on such images by including other senses, such as the tastes and smells associated with a picnic in a lake or forest scene. You can add details. You might also bring movement into the picture. For example, picture yourself swaying or dancing alone on the shore of a lake, listening to the sounds of the water, the rustle of leaves. There is no limit to what you can include, as long as the image is not distressing.

At times you may find that you can maintain one detailed image for a long time. At other times, your mind may flit from one image to another, or you may find images merging and blending. This is fine, as long as you are relaxed. There is no right way or wrong way to do this. Try to find what works best for you.

Videos, Television, and Reading

Many people use television or other video formats to tune things out. People, in general, tend to unwind in front of the television or computer screen at night. But when you spend too much time viewing things on screens, it can cease to be relaxing and become more of a substitute for living. Others become "hooked" on romance novels or mysteries and neglect sleep and/or fall into a habit of unhealthy snacking. For these reasons, we do not suggest that you should try distracting yourself all the time, but there are times when distraction can help you feel a greater sense of control, create a sense of relaxation, and reduce the intensity of your pain.

In sum, some types of distraction are passive, such as watching a show, whereas others require more action on your part, such as practicing the relaxation exercises we described earlier. Some create feelings of warmth and coziness (practicing breathing), whereas others are stimulating (for example, playing a video game). No method is better than any other or all the time. You have to find the one or ones that are most helpful for you, and you can switch around at different times.

It is important to remember that you have at least some control over the focus of your attention. It is fine to be skeptical that you will be able to distract yourself. However, it is worth your effort to try. The bottom line is that attention is a reinforcer. If you pay too much attention to everything that is not good in your relationship with your body (such as pain and circumstances related to pain), that relationship will deteriorate. Likewise, when you pay attention to everything that is good, your relationship with your body will be healthier. You may still experience pain, but you will also be empowered to care for yourself.

Creating a Pleasant and Relaxing Home Environment

In addition to creating peaceful spaces in your body, it is important to create a peaceful refuge in your home. Do you have a favorite room or a part of a room where you feel most peaceful? Are you able to set limits on family members, friends, or roommates so that you have time alone in your "space"? Think about this and how to approach significant others (if needed) to safeguard your haven for at least part of the day.

Here are some experiences our patients have reported as being refreshing and refueling as they manage their pain in their home environment:

- I nestle myself in my most comfortable chair and put on my favorite music. Sometimes I choose music that suits my mood. If I feel sad, I allow myself to listen to melancholy music. If I feel peppy, I play something lively. I really try to listen to the music. In particular, I resist the urge to do something else at the same time I am listening.

- In the evening, I take a warm bath or shower at around 8:00 p.m. Then I put on my favorite pajamas. I choose relaxing reading material. Books of meditations (for example, daily readings) and children's books are my favorites. Then I settle into a comfortable chair with good lighting and light a candle with a lavender scent. After reading for about a half hour, I am ready to go to sleep.

- I find poetry to be a great way to relax. I try to read passages in the rhythm the author intended. Sometimes I listen to poems on podcasts or CDs.

Besides alone time, many people find the company of good friends in their relaxing space to be a great solace. As several of our patients told us,

- I always seek the company of people with whom I can be my real self. I invite them over in the evening in winter, light a fire, put on soft music, and fix a pot of decaffeinated tea. With some friends, I may offer a glass of wine. Then I try to simply be present with them in the moment. If I find myself talking too much, I try to remember that listening is more relaxing than talking at these times.

- It took a while, but I finally convinced my husband to spend 15 minutes just relaxing on the couch with me. No television. Sometimes we listen to old radio programs that have been recorded—nothing stressful (like the news of today). Sometimes we just listen to music that we both enjoy. Now, my husband looks forward to our relaxing time as much as I do.

- I asked my wife to spend time with me in the evening just nestling together— no sexual demands, just tender touch and caressing. She was leery at first. But now she understands that I just want to hold her and be held. I'm not trying to set up a prelude to sex. Interestingly, though, our sex life at other times has improved as a result.

The theme of all these patients' experiences is that relaxing means not "doing" or "having" but simply "being." They also illustrate the importance of letting go of expectations and approaching each period of relaxation with an open mind and an open heart. There are no rights and wrongs, no "should" or "musts," no measures by which they rate their period of relaxation or its results. These patients have learned that despite pain, they can learn to enjoy the moment, without having to achieve anything.

Enjoying Food

Sometimes when we are in pain, we have no appetite. It is hard to even think about preparing and eating, let alone enjoying, a nutritious meal. At other times, we may use food as an anesthetic. We eat mindlessly to take our minds off our pain. Planning a nutritious meal and eating in a slow, relaxed way may seem foreign to us at those times. However, nutritious meals served in your nicest dishes, even if you are dining alone, can create a sense of peace and relaxation, as well as contributing to good health.

Maybe you use food in unhealthy ways. If you do, perhaps just once a week you can make one meal something special. Plan the menu, and set aside time to set the table to create a "dining atmosphere" (for example, you can use candles, flowers, or your favorite dishes, placemats, or tablecloth). Be creative. After you have prepared the meal, sit down and really take time to savor each bite of food. Some people find it relaxing to have some soft music in the background. Reading and texting while eating, however, tends to distract one from the pleasure of eating. If this seems too much for you right now, try doing the same with a snack of fresh fruit in the middle of the day this week.

Enjoying a relaxed meal or snack not only induces relaxation but it also aids digestion. After the meal or snack is over, take time to have decaffeinated coffee or tea. If you are alone, perhaps you can use this time to think about next week's special meal or tomorrow's snack. Even planning the meal or snack can be relaxing and can be a helpful distraction from pain. Try this for a few weeks. If you find that it relaxes you, you can increase the number of meals in which you truly enjoy your food in the weeks to come.

Enjoying Nature

Pain often gives one a feeling of being imprisoned, isolated, and alone. To decrease the feeling of being a "shut-in," try to plan an outing that is not too taxing and that involves being in a natural environment. Maybe there is a park or some woods in your area, or maybe you are fortunate enough to be near a river, lake, or even the ocean. If it is winter, dress in layers, so you can adjust to the temperature as needed. Perhaps you will only stay for 5 minutes at first. Eventually, you may find yourself staying longer.

If it is too cold or hot, perhaps you can people-watch at a mall, coffee shop, or bookstore. Some people like to just be around people without having to necessarily interact with them.

Give yourself options. Try to get out of the house at least once a day at first, even if only for a few minutes. Try this for at least a week. Then, you can adjust the frequency and length of outings to fit your particular situation.

GIVING YOURSELF ROOM TO BREATHE

What we have described so far is only part of a large number of activities that can be distracting and relaxing. Others include massage, fishing, sitting in the sun (with sunscreen or protective clothing on), or going to an outdoor cafe for a glass of iced tea in the summer. There are no limits. We list more activity ideas at the end of Lesson 4.

It's odd to think that you have to be patient to learn to "be" and to do the simplest things. But it is true. Give yourself the gift of relaxation, even if it takes a while to find what relaxes you most. The nonactivity you choose is not as important as giving yourself permission to experiment, forget your worries, and find room to breathe and get to know yourself and significant others again.

You can create your own ways of relaxing, just by practice. If you are better able to relax, despite the pain, you will have increased energy, a longer attention span, and a greater ability to concentrate. Over the course of a day, alternating what you have learned in this lesson (relaxation) with what you have learned in the previous lesson (increased activities) can improve your life immeasurably.

When you are in chronic pain, you may feel these lessons are too simple or too basic to help. You may wonder how they will help you decrease your pain. With this in mind, let's recap some of the main benefits of learning to relax:

- If your muscles are tense, you use energy that can be better spent on the things you want to do or enjoy.

- If your muscles are relaxed, you produce energy—physical, mental, and emotional.

- When you balance activity with relaxation, you learn to hear more clearly what your body is saying to you. Therefore, you will not do more than you are able to, but you will not do less.

- With the peace that comes from maintaining a proper energy balance, you become able to let go of things that are truly not in your control.

Coping with pain requires a lot of energy—mental, physical, and emotional. When activity is balanced with relaxation, you put money in your energy bank. When this equation gets out of balance, you withdraw money from the bank. Pretty soon, your account is overdrawn, and your pain levels increase. As a result, you can become oversensitive to stimuli and experience chronic fatigue and sleep problems.

When your energy account is flush, you will find that the pain or your experience of it will be less. Your immune system will be strengthened, and you will experience less fear and better concentration.

SUMMARY

- With constant and frequently recurring pain, you may feel that a battle is going in your body. You may feel you cannot fight anymore, and you cannot escape. Your body is letting you down, and you may become angry, tense, depressed, and demoralized.

- Not only these factors in yourself but also factors in your surroundings (financial problems and lack of understanding from your employer, friends, partner, children, doctor, insurance company) contribute to uncertainty and tension. Distress interferes with your ability to rest adequately and have a good night's sleep.

- Tension means that you put the muscles of your body under pressure. You are ready to fight or for flight. Your fuel is used up, and no new fuel is produced. Sooner or later, the result is exhaustion.

- Relaxation means that you free your body of pressure. You produce energy. All your muscles are in a state of deep relaxation.

- Tension demands a lot of energy. Pain, like tension, costs a lot of energy. With chronic pain, the energy (mental as well as physical) usage is high, and the energy creation is slow.

- It is not true that being healthy is an automatic result of exercise, healthy food, and sufficient fresh air. You need a balance between effort and relaxation.

- It is not true that sufficient rest and vacations automatically ensure relaxation. Relaxation means that you loosen your muscles and your thoughts.

- It is only by systematic relaxation exercises, peaceful thoughts, and the creation of a pleasant atmosphere that both the voluntary and involuntary muscles are able to relax. If you cannot arrange to accomplish this, you will soon feel burnt out and exhausted. With some practice, you can create your own sense of relaxation anywhere and at any time.

QUESTIONS TO CONSIDER

1. What are the different sources of muscle tension for you? Which muscle groups tend to get tense? When do you most often discover your muscles are tense?

2. What does doing "nothing" look like for you—for example, can it be a physical movement that calms your mind? Does it look like being physically still and stimulating your mind? What is different for you between rest, relaxation, exercise, and diversion?

3. What thoughts tend to make you more tense?

4. Thinking back in time, recently or long ago, answer the following questions:
   - Where and with whom have you been able to relax? Did you relax more alone or with others?
   - Were there certain activities (or nonactivities) that made you more relaxed?
   - Were there certain thoughts, worries, or people who interrupted your relaxation? In the same vein, were there thoughts or people who made you feel more relaxed?

 – Were there particular times of the day when you were best able to relax? Morning, afternoon, evening?

HOME ACTIVITIES

1. Make a daily schedule in which you experiment with a good balance between exertion, diversion, and relaxation. Use the charts from Lesson 2 or download a template you find online.

2. Choose a day in the week for a meal that you prepare, so you have time to enjoy it. Write down the day, the meal, and the atmosphere you will try to create.

3. Choose a day in the week for a nice breakfast. What day? What will you eat? Write this down.

4. Relaxation is a skill just like riding a bicycle or skating. It takes practice to become good at it. Try to find times when you are least likely to be disturbed. Perhaps sometime in the morning and sometime in the late afternoon or early evening would be best. Think about your day. What two times would be best for you?

5. Practice controlled breathing at least twice a day every day this week. Start with 2 minutes the first day, then add a minute each day thereafter. To track your progress, use a chart like the one provided in Figure 3.1.

FIGURE 3.1. Breathing Exercises Tracking Chart

	Day 1	Day 2	Day 3	Day 4	Day 5	Day 6	Day 7
Morning	___ min	___ min	___ min	___ min	___ min	___ min	___ min
Afternoon	___ min	___ min	___ min	___ min	___ min	___ min	___ min
Evening	___ min	___ min	___ min	___ min	___ min	___ min	___ min
Total	___ min	___ min	___ min	___ min	___ min	___ min	___ min

APPENDIX 3.1
PROGRESSIVE MUSCLE RELAXATION

Some people find it helpful to have a script for focusing while relaxing. Here is an example of one.

Close your eyes for a few moments and focus on how your body feels. Move your focus to different parts of your body and see whether you can notice any tension in any particular part. How about where you have the most pain? Can you detect any tension there? You may feel more pain when you focus on it. That's natural. You may not feel any tension at first. That is natural, as well. Just let what is "be" without judging the exercise or yourself.

If you notice tension in any part of your body, compare that sensation with body parts that don't feel as tense. Now just let the tension go, let it drift away. It might be helpful to imagine the tense body part feeling more and more like the parts of your body that do not feel tense.

Now, curl the toes of your left foot toward the bottom of your foot or the floor.

- Hold this tense position. Feel the tightness in your ankle and the sole of your foot. Note how it feels exactly.
- Now, relax your foot by moving your toes away from the bottom of your foot or the floor.
- Let your toes relax. Let the tension drain from your toes. Feel the warm, comfortable sensations of relaxation that you have been able to produce.
- Pay attention to these sensations and notice how they differ from the cramped or tight sensations of tensing your muscles.
- Pull the toes of your left foot up toward your face, and repeat the steps.
- Repeat the entire sequence with your right foot.

Continue using these instructions, replacing the first sentence with the following instructions, and alternating right to left where applicable:

Now, tense the muscles in your left [right] thigh by pressing hard against your other leg. Relax your thigh.

- Tighten the muscles of your buttocks by pulling them toward each other. Relax your buttocks.
- Tighten the muscles of your stomach as if you were trying to protect yourself from being punched. Relax your stomach muscles.
- Pull your shoulder blades toward each other. Relax your shoulder blades.
- Hunch your shoulders toward your ears. Relax your shoulders.
- Press the upper part of your right arm against your right side. Relax the upper right arm muscles. Do the same with the left arm.

APPENDIX 3.2
CONTROLLED BREATHING

Before you begin practicing, you may want to read over this exercise a few times to get familiar with it before trying it out. Some people find it helpful to record themselves reading the exercise and then playing it back. You can try different methods. We recommend that you wear loose, comfortable clothing and that you find a quiet, relaxing place to practice.

First, lie on your back. Place your hands just above your navel or "belly button." Close your eyes and imagine a balloon inside your abdomen. Each time you breathe in, imagine the balloon filling with air. Each time you breathe out, imagine the balloon collapsing.

Now inhale slowly and deeply through your nose. Let your abdomen rise as you breathe in to the count of four (for example, 4 seconds). Then, also to the count of four, exhale through your mouth, feeling your abdomen sink as you do so.

Try practicing 10 breaths, three to four times a day. Once you have been able to do this, on the next day, with each slow breath in, focus on a single word such as CALM; on the out-breath, think of a related word, such as RELAX. Some people who belong to a religion or spiritual practice find words from their faith to focus on. If none of these options appeal to you, simply repeat BREATHING IN on the in-breath and BREATHING OUT on the out-breath.

Try to stay with the words you have chosen, which may be more difficult than it seems. When your mind wanders, that's okay; gently bring it back to your word as you breathe in and out. If you are still having difficulty, try to choose a short word or shorten the word you have chosen and focus on each letter. For example, if you have chosen the word *calm*, as you breathe in, you would focus on each letter: C-A-L-M.

Once you have mastered this, you can begin to focus specifically on relaxing the muscle group that is easiest for you to relax. The next day, add another muscle group. Gradually work up to 15 minutes of controlled breathing, focusing, and relaxation. As you get better and better at this, you can try it out even when you are not sitting or lying down but are more active. In fact, some people find this exercise easier when they are stretching or slowly walking. In this way, you can take brief, mini-relaxations for a few seconds or minutes at any time.

APPENDIX 3.3
EXAMPLE OF A PLEASANT IMAGE

Read this example through, and then try to imagine yourself in this or a similar scene. It may be helpful to record yourself reading or have someone you care about make a recording for you.

Picture yourself standing by the shore of a large lake, looking out across an expanse of blue water and beyond, to the far shore. Immediately in front of you stretches a small beach and behind you a grassy meadow. The sun is shining brightly and feels very pleasant, bathing the landscape in a shimmering brightness.

It is a gorgeous spring day. The sky is pale blue, with a few soft, fluffy clouds drifting by. The breeze is blowing gently, just enough to make the trees sway and to make ripples in the grass. Feel the wind on your cheeks. You have this perfect day entirely to yourself, with nothing to do and nowhere to go.

You have a blanket, a towel, and a bottle of lemonade with you, and you carry them lightly as you walk through the meadow. You find a spot, spread the blanket, and set your lemonade aside.

Now, lie down on your blanket. It is a soft spot, and you feel comfortable. There are only a few gentle noises: a bird chirping, the breeze occasionally blowing over the meadow. The quiet is peaceful and relaxing. Tell yourself to relax and take it easy. Think about the warm, beautiful day.

Feel the sun on your body. Let go of your cares and enjoy the sensations you are feeling now.

After a while, you hear the water lapping at the shore in the distance. You take a drink of your lemonade, savoring the sour sweetness.

You walk toward the water, feeling the soft, lush grass of the meadow under your feet. You reach the sand of the beach and feel the different texture under your feet.

The sand is warm but not too warm. Let any tension remaining drain into the sand.

Now visualize yourself walking into the water slowly. Feel the refreshing wetness as the water reaches your ankles. As you feel ready, walk into the water until it is up to your knees. The sun has warmed the water pleasantly. It is almost like being in a bath.

As the breeze continues to blow gently, you look around. You have this lovely spot all to yourself.

Far across the lake, you can see a sailboat, tiny in the distance. It is so far away that you can just make out the white sail jutting up from the blue water. You stay in the water as long as you like.

When you are ready, return to your spot in the meadow. Take another drink of lemonade. Lie down and just enjoy it.

Are You Always Tired?

Ways to Combat Fatigue

Fatigue is here, in my body, in my legs and eyes. That is what gets you in the end.
—MARGARET ATWOOD, *THE HANDMAID'S TALE*

Chronic pain is usually accompanied by chronic fatigue. Many people with chronic pain report that they do not get a good night's sleep and that they doze off and on during the day. As a result, they lack energy, feel weak, and experience tiredness, even after mild exertion. So, it is not only the pain that causes you to limit your activities, but it may also be an enduring sense of fatigue and weakness.

This kind of tiredness can be every bit as disabling as the pain itself. You may drag yourself through the day. You feel as if you can't even face minor chores. Everything seems like too much. Without really meaning to, you tell everyone by your behavior, "Leave me alone."

The troubling thing is that this sense of fatigue never seems to go away, even when you are inactive and do little or nothing. Even though you believe you hear your body saying, "Take it easy, sit down, or lie down for an hour," you're not sure it's the right thing to do. You wonder whether you can trust your body at all.

In this lesson you will learn the following:

- What causes extreme fatigue and how it can be overcome;
- how your sleep, eating, and activity patterns affect your store of energy;
- how certain lifestyle habits rob you of energy; and
- what is most important in restoring your energy balance so that you can feel rested again.

Your energy system can be likened to a power generator or a battery. A generator needs fuel to create power. If there is no fuel, even the strongest generator is unable to produce power. The fuel for your body is created in tiny energy centers in your cells, called *mitochondria*. These mitochondria need a small amount of energy to be able to function adequately. Like a car battery, your "battery" can only be charged when you still have some energy in reserve.

When you are too tired, your body does not have enough energy to produce the minimal charge you need to be active. It is important, therefore, to maintain sufficient energy reserves. If you go to sleep exhausted, there will be no electrical charge to allow your battery or energy centers to operate. That is why you may wake up tired even before you begin your day.

Let's begin with a simple suggestion: Learn to know and respect your limits. As we noted in Lesson 2, a good balance of activity and rest throughout the day will ensure that there is still fuel left in reserve for your power generator to operate throughout the night. If you skipped over or skimmed Lesson 2, this might be a good time to read or review it. In Lesson 3, you learned how to tap into that deep relaxation energy by enjoying music, nature, a warm bath, and so on. Relaxation sometimes means being passive but can also involve actively focusing your attention and your breathing.

There are many kinds of tiredness. The following sections describe three kinds: emotional, physical, and nutritional.

EMOTIONAL TIREDNESS

After strenuous physical activity, it is normal to feel some fatigue. If you have worked on the suggested activities so far, you are well acquainted with this normal sense of physical tiredness. There is, however, another sort of fatigue that is often ignored—emotional tiredness. This kind of tiredness occurs when you have to do boring, uninteresting, or repetitive work. It can also occur when you are alone and isolated or when you are annoyed and frustrated. It most often occurs in relation to other people. For example, as we discuss in a later lesson, miscommunication and conflict with friends and family can create enormous emotional stress. This stress leads to emotional tiredness. Likewise, being around someone who is tiring (for example, who complains, "yes, buts," always sees the glass as half empty, or talks nonstop) is not as rewarding as sitting quietly with a friend whom you value.

Another less well-recognized cause of emotional tiredness is lack of success at what we try. It is exhausting and draining to continually feel as if one has failed or fallen short of expectations. This emotional tiredness often occurs with our chronic pain patients. When they begin becoming active and balancing rest with activity, they feel what they are doing does not amount to much. We remind them that there is a big difference between what they want to do eventually and what they can do in the present moment. Change evolves gradually if it is to last.

Do you get annoyed with yourself and your progress? Do you feel frustrated? Do you get angry with yourself when you cannot do what you want to do? Do you feel fed up with your life in general? Many of our patients do. We explain to them that this constant annoyance and scolding of oneself increases feelings of fatigue.

For many, these feelings and fatigue are too quickly linked to the amount of activity they are able to do. When gauging your progress toward your activity goals, the quality of activity may be more important than quantity. For example, gamblers can stand for hours behind a coin-operated slot machine without being bored or fatigued. Many have to virtually wrestle themselves away from the machine or go broke before they stop this repetitive action. A similar activity that required hours of standing, minus the addicting lights, noises, and feelings of hopeful anticipation that gambling provides, would be deadly boring and thus tiring. Likewise, many of us can spend hours in concentrated thought while playing computer games, scrolling our social media feeds, or texting back and forth with our friends. When faced with necessary chores we do not like, however, we can become fatigued after a relatively brief period, even if the chores are sedentary ones like sitting at a table and paying bills.

So, when considering progress, the quality, not the quantity, of activity has to be taken into consideration. Playing solitaire at the computer for 2 hours is not as qualitatively good for a person as walking for 10 or even 5 minutes. Sitting in front of the television for 2 hours is not as qualitatively successful as doing a relaxation exercise for 5 or 10 minutes.

One way to avoid this kind of emotional fatigue is to define success on your own terms. When you are resting, choose to do things that increase your self-worth or induce relaxation. When you are active, choose activities you look forward to doing with people you look forward to seeing. This is particularly important at the beginning of your efforts. Later, you can take on activities that may not initially engage you and give them a try.

Many people do not realize that these emotional factors can drain their energy and make them feel tired. You might have thought, "I do not understand why I am so tired; I have done practically nothing" or "I'm sick and tired of feeling sick and tired!" With chronic pain, emotional fatigue invariably plays a role in chronic tiredness. The less you do, the more tired you become.

PHYSICAL TIREDNESS

When you feel pain, it may affect your posture—the way you sit, stand, and move. In effect, you unconsciously adapt your posture to the pain. Pain may also make your movements slower, less coordinated, and erratic. For example, you may jerk when you don't mean to; you might move in a rigid and protected fashion.

Stop reading for a moment and become aware of how you are sitting. Are you upright or listing to one side? If you don't notice anything sitting, get up and naturally walk across a room toward a mirror. Was your movement slow or tense? Did you feel a little off balance? Were you stooped in any way or leaning to one side?

Some people who have back pain, for example, may limp slightly. The intent of limping is to protect from pain, but this distorted movement reduces strength in the affected muscles. It also places strain on the muscles that have to compensate for the awkward movement. Others who have been involved in a motor vehicle accident may have developed a whiplash disorder. To avoid pain, they hold their heads in a rigid way and reduce their neck movements. Over time, people become unaware of the restrictions or the awkwardness of their movements. Restricting or altering correct movement may reduce your pain temporarily but, over time, will lead to weakened muscles and more pain.

In almost all cases of chronic pain, people contract more muscles than may be necessary even if it does not show in the mirror. These small corrections have also been a well-intentioned effort to decrease or minimize pain. However, this, too, leads over time to more pain and greater disability.

Chronic pain may lead you to become less active over time. One consequence of inactivity is weight gain, especially around the stomach. This added weight, coupled with weakened abdominal muscles, places a strain on the back and can also cause postural changes that add to pain. Once you decrease activity, over time, you will feel increased fatigue, leading to more inactivity and more pain—a vicious revolving door that is difficult to exit.

The question, then, is not whether you should be active. The question is how much activity you should perform, for how long, and in what way. In a nutshell, that is what this lesson is about! The goal is to improve strength, endurance, and flexibility, which will, over time, lead to decreased pain. You may have found that increasing your activity level, as we suggested in Lesson 2, has increased your feelings of fatigue. This should not be a surprise because if you have been inactive for some time, your muscles are weak. However, if you gradually build up the amount of activity you perform, you will find that the increased muscle tone will allow you to do more for longer periods without a sense of exhaustion. If you have done too much after reading Lesson 2, you may feel more tired, as well. Review your charts to see whether you may have started at too high a level. Or perhaps you did not allow enough rest between periods of activity.

As we have noted several times, do not be disheartened if things are going slowly in terms of progress. This is to be expected. If you stick with your plan, even if you have had to modify it, you will begin to notice improvements in your muscle flexibility, strength, and endurance. These improvements will allow you to do more with less pain and fatigue. The improvements will occur gradually and at different rates for different people.

A benefit of becoming active and exercising is that it helps the body increase the production of internal pain-relieving chemicals. Research has demonstrated that the body produces analgesics or pain reducers that are similar to morphine and are referred to as *endorphins*. Endorphins are the body's natural pain reducers. This explains how, as you increase your activities, not only will you build up your muscular stamina but you may also experience a reduction in pain.

Many of our patients have had chronic pain for a long time. It takes time to undo the effects of inactivity and allow the body to increase its production of these natural pain reducers. As we tell our patients, be realistic. Do not expect change to occur over a few days or weeks. Stay with your activity and relaxation plans for the long haul.

NUTRITIONAL TIREDNESS

Pain, discomfort, and resulting negative moods can have different effects on people. For some of our patients, appetite disappears. For others, appetite increases. Both eating too much and eating too little have a negative influence on energy levels. How is your appetite? Do you eat three regular meals each day or six mini-meals? What about snacking of the nonnutritional kind? Have you lost or gained weight since your pain began? How much you eat can make a difference in how you feel, as can the content of your diet. Salty and sugary snack food that is low in nutritional value may be appealing, but it adds calories and, ultimately, excess weight. Thus, be aware of your eating habits (often, we snack without even paying much attention) and try to moderate the amount of food you eat that has little nutritional value and can add to your weight.

If you eat too little, it may be because food has lost its appeal over time. Or you may feel you do not have the energy needed to prepare a meal. Perhaps your pain is so severe you feel you just can't make the effort. Or perhaps you nibble snack foods throughout the day that do not require much preparation but, as noted, have little nutritional value. Even then, you may feel you have to force yourself to eat.

When you do not eat enough of the right kinds of food, you receive too little of the right kind of fuel—fuel that can turn into consistent reserves of energy. Another disadvantage of eating too little or eating the wrong foods is that the muscle tissue breaks down. Less muscle means less power and also less energy.

However, many of our patients report that their appetites increased after their pain started. When we ask them what they are eating, we learn that it is usually their "comfort foods" (candy, cookies, ice cream, salty potato chips). They want comfort because of the pain but also because they are often alone and bored. This is natural but dangerous.

For these eaters, between-meal snacks are often a particular problem. The extra calories from the snacks cause them to gain weight. If they are inactive, this weight gain often skyrockets because inactivity reduces the number of calories burned. For these inactive patients, even eating the same amount of food they ate before their chronic pain began can lead to increased weight.

And, again, another vicious circle is created: Pain leads to comfort eating (or simply eating that is now out of balance with energy burned), which leads to increased weight; increased weight leads to increased fatigue and inactivity; comfort eating begins again; and so on.

What can help? Because during the day you need energy, you should begin eating three nutritious meals (or six mini-meals) regularly. Eat as little as possible between these meals or mini-meals. If you do feel a need for snacks, try eating some fruit, raw vegetables, or a few nuts instead of cookies or potato chips. Protein from nuts, meat, and dairy products gives you long-lasting energy; fiber from fruit and vegetables helps you feel full.

Another problem all of us face is that we are often on automatic pilot when it comes to eating. As described in Lesson 3, many times, we eat without even being aware that we are eating. We taste the first bite, but space out or do other things while eating, so we don't taste much of the rest. Try eating more mindfully and slowly. Try to savor every bite. You may find that you are full on much less food this way.

If you are a comfort food eater, before turning to food, ask yourself, "What am I feeling?" Consider the following emotions: anger, irritation, frustration, sadness, disappointment or depression, grief, hopelessness, helplessness, fear, worry or anxiety, or boredom. Just recognizing which emotion you might be feeling at the moment you pick up a donut, for example, can help you make different choices and resist eating foods high in calories and with little real nutritional value.

If you still feel like snacking, ask yourself, Does this snack contain good calories? Will it provide me with an immediate "lift" only to let me down later? Will it provide me with energy, or will it simply add to my weight? Are there any substitutes that might do the trick (for example, sugar-free cocoa and whole-wheat toast with cinnamon instead of a chocolate bar)?

Finally, if you are having trouble keeping your weight down, consider eating your main meal (or mini-meals) during the middle of the day. At night, we don't require as many calories, so a light evening meal and a small nutritious "bedtime snack" (for example, a bowl of oatmeal or a cup of skim milk) may be all you need.

Our patients and readers of this book have shared with us a number of tips for overcoming nutritional tiredness and thus gaining energy:

- Eat a balanced diet. Current USDA guidelines recommend that about 50% of your daily intake be vegetables and fruits, 25% lean protein, and 25% whole grains.

- Another approach to "balancing" your diet is simply to add more of what is good to your meals. For most of us, this means adding more whole vegetables and fruits, but it may also mean to occasionally swap in a different type of protein (for example, chicken, fish, cheese, beans) than you normally consume.

- Many smart device apps are available to help you with counting calories; some also include recipe ideas and helpful articles.

- Avoid abrupt changes in your diet; lose or gain weight slowly so that you can learn how to eat to maintain your weight later. Check with your doctor before trying any special diet or eating schedule that varies significantly from the USDA guidelines (for example, keto diets, carb cycling, cutting out certain food groups entirely, intermittent fasting, weight gain smoothies, or supplements).

- For decreasing portion size, use a small plate. It's amazing the difference a small plate makes!

- Exercise before you eat to become more mindful of what your body actually needs for fuel.

- Eat slowly; savor each bite. Find a nutrition "buddy," partner, or weight-loss support group (some support groups are free).

IMPROVING SLEEP

A puzzling thing for many is that tiredness as a result of pain and fatigue does not automatically lead to deep and refreshing sleep. You may have noticed this yourself.

How would you describe your sleep? Consider the following questions: Is your sleep restless? Does your body more or less remain in a state of alarm throughout the night? Do you have problems falling asleep at night or staying asleep? Do you have bad dreams or nightmares? Does your pain wake you up during the night? If your answer to one or more of these questions is yes, you almost surely do not feel rested when you wake up.

How is your general mood during the day? Consider the following questions: Are you often irritable? Do you feel sad for no apparent reason? Do you often feel like "giving up"? Have you lost interest in activities you can still do? Do you sometimes feel "worthless"? Many people with chronic illness or chronic pain become depressed. This is not surprising. Who would not become depressed if, in addition to the daily routine of life, they had to struggle with illness or pain every day? Who wouldn't be depressed if every day they were aware of the things that they were no longer able to do?

Lack of sleep and poor sleep quality can be symptoms of depression. They can also worsen the other symptoms of depression described earlier. So, it is no surprise that when people do not get restful sleep, they often try prescribed or over-the-counter sleeping pills. Others turn to alcohol as a way of getting to sleep or staying asleep and avoiding feeling depressed. Unfortunately, these remedies, if used for more than 2 weeks, can actually worsen the sleep problem. Sleep medication or alcohol may lead to light sleep throughout the night so that when you awaken, you notice that a number of hours have passed, but you still feel tired. Many of these drugs (yes, as noted, alcohol is a drug) create dependency if used daily over even a short period. And they do not solve the sleep problem; they only temporarily mask the symptoms.

Changing thoughts and behaviors can improve some symptoms of depression, and in a later lesson, we offer help with that. But for now, let's continue with our discussion of sleep.

It is important to know that the amount of sleep you get and the quality of that sleep are not the same. In general, there is a light stage of sleep and a deep sleep, in which dreaming often occurs. It is this deep sleep that is truly refreshing.

Our highest hope for you to improve sleep and your overall state of well-being is that you develop the conviction that you can manage your level of pain and yourself. Say it: I can manage myself. The program described in this book, followed consistently and resolutely, will give you that feeling of self-confidence, which should lead to a gradual but steady improvement in sleep patterns.

The following are a number of things you can do to achieve the deepest levels of sleep. Some of these may be familiar to you already.

- Cut back on your caffeine during the day. Caffeine, as most people know, is a stimulant. That is why so many people "need" a cup of coffee to get them going in the morning (they also "need" it because their bodies become physically dependent on caffeine).

- Even people who know that caffeine arouses them may not know that caffeine, even if consumed early in the day, can interfere with sleep. We don't suggest that you go off caffeine "cold turkey." First, keep a log of how many drinks you have each day. Gradually cut back (for example, cut out one caffeinated beverage one day, cut out that one and a second the next, and so on).

- Cut back on alcohol and do not consume alcohol past 7:00 in the evening.

- Design your own personalized bedtime ritual. The human body likes a fixed rhythm and regularity. Sleep rituals involve consistently following the same steps before you go to bed. For example, some of our patients lay out their sleep clothes, read a meditation or other comforting short passage, and take a warm bath before they go to bed. Another option is to go into another room and do something that is not too interesting, stimulating, or exciting for a half hour.

- Keep a neat and comfortable bedroom. Change linens at least once a week, buy supportive pillows, choose a firm (not too hard or soft) mattress that does not squeak.

- Adjust temperature and light. The environment in which you sleep is also important. Rooms that are too warm or too cold can hinder sleep. Too much light can also be a problem. That includes light from cell phones and computers, so turning them off or placing them in another room might be helpful.

- Exercise close to bedtime (2–3 hours before you go to sleep).

- Go to bed and get up at a fixed time, even if you have slept poorly the previous night. This will help you stay consistent with your routine.

- Avoid naps during the day. Naps may seem natural when you have not slept well the night before, but they often interfere with sleep at night.

- If you cannot drop off to sleep, or if you lie awake at night, alternate up and down time. Get out of bed after 20 minutes, and even if you do not feel sleepy, go back to bed after 30 minutes. If you still do not get sleepy after 20 minutes, repeat this ritual. Remember not to do any "arousing" activities (for example, watching television, listening to the radio, surfing the Internet) or think about worrisome topics when you are up. For the first week or so, you may feel somewhat tired during the day, but your body and mind will gradually learn that you mean business when it comes to sleep. Keep with this pattern until you can fall asleep and stay asleep for the entire night.

- When not asleep in bed at night, relax your muscles. Even if you do not fall asleep, lying relaxed will help you feel better. If you fall asleep in a relaxed manner, you will feel much more rested. You might find this a good time to review some of your pleasant mental images (see Lesson 3 for suggestions).

- There are smartphone apps designed to support sleep and provide relaxing music and gentle instructions for guiding your thoughts and breathing.

Although doing things on this list will help, be aware that just as you cannot force relaxation, you cannot force sleep. You can, however, create the conditions for a good night's sleep and do so consistently.

A (NECESSARY) RETURN TO PACING

Pacing is so important that although we have covered it in Lesson 2, we want to stress it here as well. A pattern of overactivity followed by exhaustion and pain most often leads to poor sleep. For example, if you are overactive one day and underactive the next, the following night, you are unlikely to sleep well. The body loves consistent and healthy patterns. Taking breaks from activity on schedule, rather than when you are exhausted, is a good pattern. Getting up and being active on schedule, rather than when you feel like it, is a good pattern as well. As mentioned earlier, some of our patients buy an inexpensive kitchen timer to remind them when a period of rest or activity is scheduled to occur. This kind of balance gradually builds into a serene and healthy lifestyle that decreases pain and increases enjoyment.

We call this "balanced growth," as illustrated in Figure 4.1. Staying between the dotted lines (optimal level of activity) means growth, success, and energy. Too much or too little activity means setbacks, anxiety, failure, and fatigue.

FIGURE 4.1. Balanced Growth

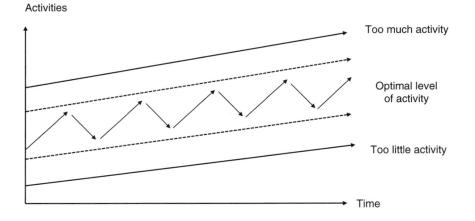

Remember, the pattern of resting before becoming excessively tired is not laziness. It is healthy pacing that allows you to have energy in reserve. During a break from activity, you should plan to do something pleasant and relaxing, something that you enjoy. It's best to determine before your activity period what it is you want to do when you rest.

Regularity is the key to pacing. Skipping a break to try to do more or skipping activity when you want to do nothing often leads to a loss in the ability to be active when you most want to be. Moreover, this kind of irregularity can often increase pain and interfere with sleep.

In the beginning, however, it is important to experience success. So, choose relaxing activities and more energetic activities for periods you can handle. Increase these gradually, so that you can be energized by improvement.

ARE YOUR EXPECTATIONS REALISTIC?

Many of our patients observe that they need to rest for a rather long period after they first start exerting themselves. They consider this to be abnormal ("After all, I'm not 99!"). These thoughts bring up all kinds of distressing feelings—shame, guilt, sadness, frustration. You may feel this as well. What you were able to do in the past was what you considered a decent level of exertion followed by a brief period of rest and recovery.

Your typical day in the past went like this: You woke rested, carried on a number of activities during the day, rested at the end of the day, and finally, went to sleep. This activity–rest cycle most likely became connected to your feelings of success, your sense of self-worth, and your level of confidence. You may not have been aware of this at the time because you considered it normal.

When you begin to experience chronic pain, this "normal pattern" may be disrupted entirely or at least in large part. When this occurs, or if you try to push yourself back into your earlier pattern too soon, the result will likely be feelings of failure, loss of self-esteem, and diminished confidence. Nevertheless, old habits die hard. If you get up each morning resolving to achieve your old activity pattern, by evening, you will likely feel dejected and as if you have "failed."

The pattern shown at the top of Figure 4.2, however, may no longer describe your life. Even so, each morning, you get up unconsciously and automatically with the resolution still to try to achieve your old activity pattern. You do not want to accept the new realities of your life because admitting that your activity pattern has to change brings with it a strong feeling of failure and having fallen short of your expectations.

When you aim for the activity pattern shown at the top of Figure 4.2 and end up with the activity pattern shown in the middle, you may feel frustrated or afraid or experience a loss of self-respect. As soon as you feel a bit better, you are so happy and hopeful that you immediately want to return to your old pattern as often and as long as possible. You are too ashamed to admit that you no longer do as much as you used to do or would like to do. A person believes what he or she wants to believe and adapts reality to fit the belief. You consider your current activity pattern abnormal because you may feel that your battery is run down after even minor activities.

A more appropriate pattern of activity for people who have chronic pain is one such as that shown at the bottom of Figure 4.2. Here activity (white bands) and relaxation (gray bands) are coupled so that a pattern is established that helps you not to overdo it but also to keep active. Such a pattern should contribute to improved sleep and prevent excessive fatigue. It is important for you to pace your activities and to look at the division of exertion and relaxation in your daily program.

You may find it hard to accept where you are right now. This is okay, too. Acceptance takes time and patience. But it's hard to move from where you

FIGURE 4.2. Patterns of Activity

The old pattern before chronic pain, resulting in high sense of self-worth, satisfaction, and confidence:

14 hours	10 hours
ACTIVITY	REST AND SLEEP

The new normal with chronic pain, resulting in shame, anger, and depression:

2 hours	22 hours
ACTIVITY	INACTIVITY, POOR-QUALITY REST AND SLEEP

A paced approach between activity and relaxation, resulting in confidence, pain reduction, and better sleep:

2 hours	2 hours	2 hours	3 hours	2 hours	3 hours	1 hour	10 hours
Activity	Relax	Activity	Relax	Activity	Relax	Activity	REST

are to where you want to go until you begin to accept what has happened as the result of your pain. You may have to grieve these losses in ability to be active to accept them and move on.

Part of why people push themselves too hard is that they begin to increase their activity level, feel happy and hopeful, and try to return to their earlier levels of activity immediately. For these people, acceptance of their current limitations may be one of the most difficult tasks they face. However, acceptance and intentional pacing can lead to more consistent days of higher self-esteem, feelings of greater success, and more pain reduction.

DIVERSION, PRIORITIES, AND CONTROL

Although some of these topics have been or will be discussed in more detail in other lessons, we would like you to consider them here with regard to combating your chronic fatigue.

Diversion

In addition to pacing, the diversion activities described in Lesson 3 bear repeating in terms of chronic fatigue and sleep problems. A change of scenery, getting out of a rut, or doing something nice (alone or with others) gives us a boost. Journaling, painting, drawing, sewing, quilting, collecting things, enjoying nature, having a weekend away, watching a good film, reading an interesting book, and watching an exciting TV series can all be useful distractions. Beware of perfectionism if you are undertaking artistic pursuits because this can add stress to your life.

Priorities

When you're in chronic pain, it's easy to lose sight of priorities. But it is helpful to give what attention you can to those things that deserve it—the truly important things in life. For different people, this means different things. For some, it means family; for others, it means friends; and for still others, it means the ability to pursue some hobby or creative outlet. By *creative outlet*, we do not mean painting the Sistine Chapel. Cooking a delicious and beautifully presented meal is creative. Arranging a vase of flowers with your full attention is a creative act.

What is important to you now? What has been important to you in the past? What was "worth the trouble" to do before your pain began? Who was important to stay in contact with? Setting priorities is important for people with chronic pain and fatigue because energy is more limited for them than for people without pain.

What are your time-wasters or energy-drainers—certain people, certain thoughts, or mindless television or dwelling on the past? These all consume precious energy. Prioritize them out of your life.

If you are still working inside or out of the home, you may believe that hard and long hours of work are important. But most people realize at least at retirement or the end of their lives that work has not been that important.

Financial concerns are quite commonly experienced by people with chronic pain. It may be necessary to prioritize your expenses or even seek assistance from family and friends. Community resources, including civic groups, religious institutions, and charitable organizations, may provide useful support. The American Chronic Pain Association website provides a resource guide listing organizations that can help you pay for treatments your insurance plan does not cover: https://www.theacpa.org/pain-management-tools/resources/life-resources/. Some government websites, such as http://Medicare.gov, also provide information about available resources, such as pharmaceutical companies' patient assistance programs or state health insurance assistance programs.

Don't be ashamed if you have financial hardship. It is not what you have but who you are that counts. It may be helpful to share your concerns with those whom you trust and ask for advice and help from them.

When you ask children, "What do you value most in your parents?" or when you ask adults, "As a child, what did you consider your parents' best attribute?" the answer is never, "They kept the house clean and worked hard at the office." Nor is it, "They worked hard so that we could have lots of money." The answer that is more common in happy families is, "They had time for me," "They showed interest in me," "They listened to me and truly got to know me." These are important things to ponder not only with regard to others but also with regard to yourself.

How much of your time is spent showing interest in your whole self, not just your pain? How often do you truly listen to your heart? How well do you know yourself?

Control

Another energy drainer is trying to control things that are not under your control. For example, you cannot control the physical limitations associated with the causes of your pain, the weather, or how others will respond to a request. However, if you put your energy into things that you have some control over, with practice (for example, pacing, nutrition, acceptance, perseverance, and patience), you will feel more successful, hopeful, and energetic. Your pain will likely become easier to bear.

We began Lesson 1 with the Serenity Prayer: "Grant me the serenity to accept the things I cannot change, courage to change things I can, and wisdom to know the difference." Listening to other people's stories about choosing to control what is in their power to control—for example, in a support group setting—may help.

SUMMARY

- Chronic pain is usually accompanied by chronic fatigue. Everything feels as if it is too much for you. When you are too tired and exhausted, your energy system does not function as it should.

- Your fatigue may be the result of emotional, physical, and nutritional factors. Physical fatigue results from
  - inactivity and changes in your movement that cause reduced strength,
  - problems with sleeping,
  - lack of pacing of energy, and
  - bad eating habits.

  Emotional fatigue results from
  - feeling helpless, frustrated, and anxious;
  - focusing on loss and limitations;
  - having too few diversions;
  - having no clear priorities; and
  - having a lack of acceptance.

- Acceptance of chronic pain and fatigue means being open to trying new avenues to feeling better. This includes a systematic approach to increasing body movement and exercise and putting a focus on success experiences.

- Optimal activity and pacing are essential, as is keeping a balance between doing too much and too little. Over time, the amount you can exercise should increase, and the time needed to recover should get shorter.

QUESTIONS TO CONSIDER

1. What kind of activities robs you of your energy, and what kind of activities gives you energy?

2. What kind of persons robs you of your energy, and what kind of persons gives you energy?

3. How will you improve your sleeping patterns?

4. How will you improve your eating habits?

5. What does acceptance look like for you? Consider describing this in terms of what you used to consider disappointments and successes and what you consider to be disappointments and successes now. Or consider listing the things that are within your control and the things that are outside your control.

HOME ACTIVITIES

1. If you are having trouble sleeping, keep a sleep and caffeine diary. Begin by recording the time you go to sleep at night and estimating how long it takes you (approximately) to fall asleep each night. If you nap, write down how many naps you take, when you took them, and how long they lasted. Keep track of the amount and times you consume drinks or food with caffeine. How many times a week do you spend in bed doing activities other than sleeping or participating in sexual intimacy? These facts will give you a baseline from which to work.

2. Keep a food diary for 2 days. Record everything you eat and drink, including snacks and when you ate them. In your notebook or journal, describe how tired you were before and after eating each meal or snack. If you don't see a pattern emerging after 2 days, record data for several more days.

3. Make a list of your top five priorities in life (for example, grandchildren, finances, hobbies, religion).

4. Choose a time-consuming task you have been putting off and plan how you can gradually complete this task by pacing it over a week or two.

5. Make a list of the pleasurable activities you no longer do because of your pain. Then, review the following list of pleasurable activities and list five you would like to do and think you could do, despite your pain. Now put a circle around the two activities that you will try to do over the next week and get started.

SOME EXAMPLES OF PLEASANT ACTIVITIES

Spending time outdoors
Watching a sporting event
Talking to someone about sports
Going to a movie or library
Going to a museum
Planning a short trip or vacation
Buying something for yourself or others
Going to be near the water
Doing artwork
Reading the Bible
Reading a book
Playing golf (even a few holes)
Rearranging things in your house
Going to a bar or pub
Going to a restaurant
Going to a lecture
Going for a drive in the country
Writing poems
Knitting or sewing
Seeing friends
Visiting or receiving a visit from family or friends
Going camping
Having lunch with a family member or friend
Spending time with a pet
Spending time with your children, grandchildren, nieces, or nephews
Going to religious services
Going to a service, civic organization, or social club

Playing a musical instrument

Canning, freezing, or making preserves

Making food or crafts to give away or sell

Playing pool or billiards

Playing chess or checkers

Going on social media sites

Visiting friends or family who are sick

Watching birds or animals

Working in your garden

Visiting a garden

Going to a zoo or aquarium

Going to a casino

Listening to the sounds of nature

Having a lively conversation

Listening to the radio or a podcast

Getting a massage or back rub

Going on a picnic or barbecue

Buying something for a family member

Walking in the woods or mountains or by the sea or lake

Going fishing

Going to a health club or sauna

Learning to do something new

Talking on the telephone

Joining or connecting online with a self-help group

Cooking a meal

Writing in a diary

Saying prayers

Playing a board game (for example, Monopoly, Scrabble)

Playing ping-pong

Going swimming

Starting a new project

Going bird watching

Going people-watching at a park or shopping mall

Repairing something

Writing letters

Caring for house plants

Taking a walk

Beginning to collect something

Going to a garage sale

Doing volunteer work

Making a new friend or calling an old one

Traveling with a group

Going to a play

Teaching something to someone

Copying your recipes for others

Going on a nature walk

Don't Let Pain Ruin Your Relationships!

For beautiful eyes, look for the good in others; for beautiful lips, speak only words of kindness; and for poise, walk with the knowledge that you are never alone.

—AUDREY HEPBURN

There is no need to tell you that living with chronic pain can be overwhelming. It feels like it takes over your life completely and consumes all your energy. However, convincing others, including health care providers, of the impact of chronic pain and having to deal with the lack of understanding and outright skepticism is just an added burden to your life.

There is a great deal of ignorance about the topic of pain. If all pain is looked at as being a temporary and easily corrected problem, it can be hard to find understanding. Many types of chronic pain do not go away on their own and may get worse. This is a frightening problem. In this lesson, you will learn ways to talk about your pain with others. Specifically, you will learn about the impact of chronic pain on other people and how to recognize the patterns that others' responses often fall into. You will also learn ways to improve your communication and assert yourself. Finally, you will learn how to create a supportive environment around yourself.

THE IMPORTANCE OF COMMUNICATION

As you know by now, many people are uninformed about pain. They often assume that pain, although unpleasant, is temporary. They also believe that it will, within a brief time, be easily treated or simply go away on its own. By extension, they may believe a number of things that are false about you. For example, they may think you are not really feeling pain, you don't follow

89

doctor's orders, you are complaining to get attention, you are trying to avoid some undesirable activity, or you are trying to obtain disability payments or medications that can make you feel better. When you report chronic pain, you may feel afraid that others will consider you a complainer and think of you as being weak or a "wimp."

Many of our patients believe that the people around them think one or more of these things. Have you experienced such reactions? Have responses by others made you feel misunderstood, lonely, distressed, frustrated, angry, or some combination of these emotions? This would be hardly surprising.

Other people may say well-meaning things, but their words may inadvertently make things worse. "Give it time," one may say. But you have already given it lots of time. "You need to see another doctor," a second suggests. But you have already seen three doctors. "Have you tried one of those new drugs I saw advertised on TV?" a third asks. These kinds of suggestions or questions sometimes make you wish that everyone would just leave you alone.

However, there are times you don't want to be left alone. Living with chronic pain can be a lonely experience. You may feel abandoned by others. You may wish for emotional support, especially when the pain is at its worst. And you do need help with some things at some times. If only they knew how hard it was for you to ask!

On their first visit to our offices, many of our patients tell us that their lives now revolve around their bed, lounge chairs, electronic devices, doctors' offices, clinics, and pharmacies. They feel lonely, isolated, and stuck in a rut. Does this describe your situation? If yes, how does it make you feel?

The likelihood of feeling isolated in this situation is greater if you feel you have no one with whom you can freely share your feelings and know that they are not judging you. Perhaps you find it hard to express yourself. Perhaps you attach great value to your independence and don't want to admit that you need support. Or perhaps there is no one around who truly understands.

Communicating Well Helps You Avoid Isolation

But consider this. Friends and family members can feel excluded, powerless, and frustrated if you do not communicate your feelings to them in an open way—a way in which they can truly hear you. If you cannot clearly express your feelings and accurately describe what you need from them, it is hard for them to know how to support you. How would you like them to help and respond to you? They can't read your mind.

In all relationships, it is the quality, not the quantity, of communication that determines whether people become distant and defensive or whether bonds are strengthened and deepened. The more people skillfully share each other's lives, desires and longings, worries and uncertainties, the greater their mutual satisfaction. This kind of communication may be difficult for you if you haven't first thought about what you need for yourself.

If you can openly and directly express what you do need and what you do not need, first to yourself and then to others, and if you let family and friends know that they can play a meaningful and important role in your recovery, you have a real chance at gaining support, affection, and encouragement. Most important, you will not feel so alone. The feelings of safety and security that result make pain easier to bear for everyone. For you living with chronic pain, these feelings reduce stress, help you get important needs met, and thus can actually decrease pain. Even when pain is at its worst, feeling safe and secure through trust and understanding makes the pain easier to bear.

To begin, consider the experience of one of our patients with regard to how chronic pain affected her relationships with other people.

Janet's Story

Janet is a 46-year-old woman who has experienced 3 years of severe and persistent pain following a car accident in which she was rear-ended. She initially sustained a whiplash injury characterized by neck and upper shoulder pain and stiffness that was treated with rest, heat, immobilization with a soft cervical (neck) collar, and pain medications. But the pain diminished very little and has now spread from her neck to multiple areas of her body. She has recently been diagnosed with fibromyalgia—that is, chronic widespread pain and a number of other physical, cognitive, and emotional symptoms.

Among her many symptoms, Janet reports frequent headaches, tingling in her fingers and toes, difficulty sleeping, trouble concentrating, and chronic fatigue. She reports that almost any activity makes her pain worse.

Janet's pain has been severe enough to disrupt all aspects of her life: family, work, social, and recreational, as well as physical. Her pain does not permit her to get a good night's sleep. Consequently, she never feels rested and is tired most of the time.

Janet acknowledges that since her injuries, she has not had time for her husband, Glenn, and her teenage children, Jamal and Tahisha. Her house is no longer as neat and tidy as it used to be.

Glenn was initially sympathetic but now says he is fed up with her constant complaints and unpredictable emotional outbursts. The expenses of her medication and medical treatments have drained the family's finances. This has meant giving up family vacations and other pleasurable activities. They are unable to afford to go out to restaurants or movies as they used to do. Glenn says this wouldn't be so bad, but Janet has no interest in any previously enjoyed activities or even in sex. She just wants to be "left alone."

Janet's children are troubled by her behavior, as well. They feel that she has become a different person since the accident. They are anxious about her unpredictable behavior and mood swings. They feel discouraged by her lack of progress toward being "their old mom."

When the children are around Janet, they are extremely solicitous, bringing her snacks, coffee, and medication; rubbing her neck; and doing whatever she asks. Inside, though, they are angry. Janet bosses them around, demanding they do whatever she asks, all because of her pain. At times, she belittles them for no apparent reason. No matter how well or quickly they do the housework, it never seems to meet her standards. They then feel they cannot do anything that will please her. They will never be "good enough" for the injured Janet.

At the time Janet and her family came for a consultation, the teenagers were confused and angry, and they had begun to stay away from home as much as possible. At the same visit, Janet acknowledged that she was angry with them because they avoid her. She accused them of not caring. She then began to cry, admitting that she feels sad and guilty about her words and behavior.

Glenn, a plumbing supplies salesman, has also recently been spending more and more time away from home, often volunteering for extended selling trips. His inaccessibility has led to greater anger on Janet's part. The continual conflicts have driven Glenn even further away, and he has had some fleeting thoughts about getting a divorce.

At the time we first saw Janet, her pain and other symptoms were consuming her energy and her life and the lives of her family.

Unfortunately, Janet's story is all too common. Living with chronic pain not only causes the patient to suffer but also affects every member of the family.

Are you aware of the impact of your pain on others? Have you noticed how their behavior affects what you think, how you feel, and what you do? What advice would you have for Janet? What would you say to Glenn and the children?

SHARING WITH FAMILY AND FRIENDS

There is an old expression: "A sorrow shared is a sorrow halved." Living successfully means sharing both the good times and the bad. The more people share in each other's lives, the greater the likelihood their relationships will bring mutual fulfillment.

When one family member has chronic pain, this kind of sharing and mutual involvement becomes more difficult. The couple or family can no longer do the things they used to do together. Time and money spent on visits to the doctor and treatments take the place of time and money for dinners out and movies.

We tell our patients that they first have to think about how they can make up for the lack of time spent with their families and friends. We emphasize the importance of *quality time*. We teach them to use their time together wisely, communicating interest and attention with words and actions. Many of our patients have closed themselves off from others, however, especially if their pain is long-standing. It takes time and courage to open up again.

How about you? Do you feel that you do not want to "burden" others with your problems? Do you want understanding and support from others but are afraid or embarrassed to have to ask for help? Do you like to give but have difficulty receiving? When you have done a great deal for others, do you feel especially let down when you get little in return? Do you find yourself being irritable with others, barking orders when you cannot bear to ask for things?

Do you act as though all is well and hide your feelings until a final drop causes the bucket to overflow? Does the straw that broke the camel's back lead you to let out all your emotions in one burst?

If you answered "yes" to any of these questions, you have likely built a wall to protect yourself. This need to protect yourself is understandable, but you may also be harboring a deep longing for others to break down these walls that you have created. When they don't, you may feel that you have to protect yourself even more.

Your family and friends are likely confused and, at times, hurt by your behavior (for example, a sudden outburst of emotion). It is likely that, like Janet, you feel ashamed, confused, and hurt after an outburst as well.

You may then seek to get yourself back in control of your feelings, to hold them within yourself. Others may not dare to discuss what has happened. Like you, they try to act as if nothing is wrong. Few people know how to handle so many intense and confusing feelings, either in themselves or others. (Remember how Janet's family responded to her?) Your friends and family may feel as inadequate and helpless as you do at times. They may not know how to respond and how to be supportive. They can't read your mind to determine what you think, want, or need from them.

Most people hope that problems in relationships will disappear on their own. The problem is, they never do. The only way to solve this problem is to learn to communicate better.

DECODING COMMUNICATION PROBLEMS

What are some common problems in communication? Most problems communicating involve one or a combination of four main issues. First, there can be a mismatch between what you say and what you want to say. For example, you might say you want everyone to go away when what you really need is either comfort or just a little bit of time to yourself. Another common problem is not knowing how to make requests for help. Asking for help is sometimes hard. You may communicate passively—for example, through body language—and deny your feelings, even to yourself. Or you may communicate aggressively and defensively, inadvertently hurting others' feelings and not respecting their needs. Third, you might have difficulty actively following and listening for context about what others are trying to communicate. You may listen but not really *hear* what is being said. Finally, are you sometimes making excessive demands, emphasizing your dependency, or even acting dishonestly? When you are in pain, you may think that people close to you *should* understand how you feel, *should* know what you want, or *should* know what to do. When they don't, you may become unreasonable and try to control them.

However, asking why others are not sensitive to your pain is a reasonable question. It may help to think about the following barriers to effective communication about pain.

Chronic Pain Is Invisible

You may look quite healthy outwardly but feel miserable on the inside. The inconsistency between appearances and feelings makes communication especially complicated.

For example, as a result of your pain, you may have a number of limitations. This has consequences for other people in your life, who need to know about them. If you look fine, other people will automatically assume that your pain is not so bad or at least is getting better. So, you have to tell them clearly what your limitations are. Particularly in the case of chronic pain, people may have to be told more than once what you are able and not able to do.

It Is Difficult for People to Know What They Should or Should Not Do

People may seem insensitive because it is difficult for them to know what they should or should not do, when to offer help, and when to back off. Men, in particular, may be confused about this. In modern society, most men have been socialized not to notice when others need help. They often do not want to notice when they need help themselves.

It Is Difficult to Imagine That Pain Will Never End

In the case of pain, particularly chronic pain, it's hard to put yourself in the shoes of another. This is because pain is personal and also because most people's experience with pain is with temporary injuries. Unless they have experienced chronic pain, it is truly incomprehensible to them that pain can have such a great impact on your life.

Other People's Pain Is Not Interesting!

You may feel left out of things because of your pain. Some days you wish you could make someone understand exactly what the pain feels like. However, many people are not naturally predisposed to hearing about this. Although it's frustrating when the other person doesn't seem interested in your pain, the hard fact of life is that pain is not that interesting unless it's happening to you! It helps not to take this personally. When people are uninterested in your pain, it does not mean that they're not interested in you. And let's face it, they likely would not be interested in anyone else's pain either.

Other People Have Their Own Problems

Many people do not wear their hearts on their sleeves. They may be preoccupied with their own problems, but they do not often admit this. Even in a marriage, people may not share their worries. Some have been taught not to talk about a problem until they have it solved. Also, many believe that they have to solve others' problems in a concrete way. If they can't fix it, they often don't know what to do. As a result, they may feel inadequate and help-less. Their role has often been the nurturer who is attuned to and takes care of others' needs. Most people don't realize that simply listening to another is perhaps the greatest source of comfort there is.

A related issue is that when you share your feelings of sadness, fear, or frustration, they may arouse others' feelings of the same sort (for example, worry over financial or work problems, sadness over an elderly parent's ill health). If other people do not want their emotions to be touched by a discus-sion of yours, they may change the topic. If you continue to talk about your pain or associated emotions, they may distance themselves physically or emo-tionally from the conversation.

Pain Is a Difficult Topic to Discuss

People usually like to avoid difficult topics, even if they have nothing negative going on in their lives, and physical pain is a difficult topic (as is dying or being unemployed). People may also think if they talk about your pain, it will only make things worse. Again, if you continue talking about it, they may tend to back away. But this has more to do with them than with you.

Pain Is Not Constant

You likely have noticed that some days your pain is somewhat better, and other days it is much worse, although it may never be completely gone. People outside the home, however, tend to see you when things are going well and not when you are stuck in the house because of the pain. When people see you during an easy day, they may quickly assume that you must be "better." You, however, know and possibly fear that there will be more challenging days ahead, so you may feel a certain reluctance to tell others that you are feeling somewhat better. You are afraid that this will give you, as well as your family and friends, false hopes and expectations. These antic-ipations can influence what you think and feel and do. We will return to this important issue later in Lesson 7.

Pain Is Unpredictable

Pain, as you know, does not always follow immediately after overexertion. It can be delayed, which is confusing to other people. They see you being busy, and then a day or so later, you are unable to do much at all. They are not sure what to expect from you. Only after they learn about the ups and downs of living with chronic pain can they understand. However, they may not be ready to learn this until you establish better communication with them. Also, pain makes it difficult to plan ahead. People close to you may feel frustrated because they can never be quite sure what type of day you are likely to have, and they, therefore, can't plan anything that includes you. People like to give to people they care about, and not being able to plan an outing for you may be as frustrating for them as it is for you.

Pain Causes Negative Feelings

As we have noted, pain, fatigue, and limitations all produce negative emotions. Sometimes you give the message, "Help me—don't you see that I'm having a difficult time?" while in an exactly comparable situation, you may spitefully say, "Don't help me—let me take care of myself. Do you think I can't do anything anymore?" Think back—how did Janet feel about her family's responses to her?

As we have illustrated, pain is a complicated topic that is difficult to understand, not only by you but also by significant people in your life. It is a topic that most people would rather avoid.

IMPROVING COMMUNICATION

Because of these difficulties in understanding chronic pain, learning to communicate well with others is particularly important. Most people have not been directly taught to communicate well, and most of the time, they "get along" pretty well anyway. However, when difficulties arise, problems in communication make things even worse. So, if you have chronic pain, it is important to learn to be an excellent communicator.

To begin this process, we have summarized a few basic guidelines for improving communication:

- Tell others respectfully what you can and cannot do.

- Let them know that the severity of your pain varies, even if it is never completely gone.

- Tell them in a friendly way what kind of help you hope to receive and why.

- Tell them when their efforts to help are successful or when you notice they are trying to help! Praise wins over blame every time.

- Do not be afraid to tell people when things are a bit better or a bit worse.

- Try to be positive, despite the pain. A pleasant disposition can sometimes decrease pain at the same time it brings others closer to you.

- Ask for understanding with regard to your difficult feelings about the pain and its consequences.

- Give a short answer to the question "How are you feeling?" Then show interest by inquiring how the other person is doing, as well.

- Talk to others regularly, not just when your pain is most intense.

- Do not have an important discussion, make rash statements, or make important decisions when your pain is at its worst.

- Try not to use body language to indirectly communicate pain (for example, grimacing, moaning, or sighing to gain attention). Try to be direct and honest in telling people how you are feeling. Encourage others to express their feelings and discuss them with you.

- Do not feel guilty if the pain has a negative influence on your moods; this is normal. Try not to take out your negative feelings on other people, however.

- Work on accepting your present limitations while making efforts to improve.

- Do not take the other person's mildly negative behavior personally. Others' moods most often reflect their personality or concerns.

Giving and Getting Respect

In addition to these guidelines, it is important to understand the nature of giving and receiving respect. For example, lashing out or engaging in arguments that hurt or anger you or others may damage mutual respect. Expressing yourself appropriately and assertively is one way to address this problem.

Assertion involves standing up for personal rights and expressing your thoughts, feelings, and beliefs in direct, honest, and appropriate ways. The basic messages when you are communicating assertively are the following: "This is what I think," "This is what I feel," "This is what I would like to happen." These messages express who you are, how you see the problem, and what you want to do about it. If they are communicated appropriately, they do not shame, humiliate, or put you or other people down.

Two types of respect are involved in assertive communication: respect for oneself and respect for the other person. The following is an example of assertive communication.

Tirzah was desperately trying to get a flight to Kansas City to see her mother, who was sick in the hospital. Weather conditions were bad, and the lines were long. Having been rejected from three standby flights, Tirzah again found herself in the middle of a long line for the fourth and last flight to Kansas City that night. This time she approached a man who was standing near the beginning of the line and said, pointing to her place, "Would you mind exchanging places with me? I ordinarily wouldn't ask, but it's extremely important that I get to Kansas City tonight to be with my mother, who is very ill." The man nodded yes.

When asked what her reaction would have been if the man had refused, Tirzah replied, "I would have been disappointed, but it would have been okay. I hoped he would understand, but after all, he was there first."

In this example, Tirzah showed self-respect by asking whether the man would be willing to help her. Also, she respected the man's right to refuse her request and not fulfill her need.

Assertion, Nonassertion, and Aggression

There are three ways to communicate with other people: assertively, non-assertively, and aggressively.

Assertion is not simply a way of getting what one wants. The goal of assertion is clear communication and mutuality—to give and receive respect, play fair, and leave room for compromise. In the case of compromise, neither person sacrifices the basic integrity of their needs.

Nonassertion involves violating one's integrity by failing to express honest feelings, thoughts, and beliefs. For example, nonassertion is expressing one's thoughts and feelings in an apologetic and overly self-effacing manner. It results in others not taking your needs seriously and may reflect that you don't take your needs seriously either.

Nonassertion also sometimes shows a subtle lack of respect for the other person's ability to shoulder some responsibility and to refuse requests appropriately. Ultimately, the goal of nonassertion is to appease others and avoid conflict. Perhaps when you exercise nonassertion, you see yourself as being a good person; however, the other may see it as an indication of weakness or even license to cross a boundary with you that they would not with someone else.

Aggression involves insisting on one's rights in a way that is inappropriate and almost always violates the rights of the other person. The goal of aggression is to dominate and win. Tactics include humiliating and belittling or overpowering people so they are less able to express and defend their needs and rights.

Table 5.1 summarizes the differences between assertive, nonassertive, and aggressive communication.

TABLE 5.1. Comparing Nonassertive, Assertive, and Aggressive Behavior

	Nonassertive	Aggressive	Assertive
Characteristics of the behavior	Emotionally dishonest, indirect, self-denying, inhibited	Inappropriate, direct, self-enhancing at expense of another, expressive	Appropriate, emotionally honest, direct, self and other enhancing, expressive
Your feelings when you engage in this behavior	Hurt, anxious at the time and possibly angry later	Righteous, superior, maybe satisfied at the time but possibly guilty later	Confident, self-respecting at the time and later
The other person's feelings about him- or herself when you engage in this behavior	Guilty or superior	Hurt, humiliated, angry	Valued, respected
The other person's feelings about you when you engage in this behavior	Pity, irritation, disgust	Anger, vengefulness	General respect

HOW OTHERS COMMUNICATE WITH THEIR BEHAVIOR

Your spouse, partner, child, or best friend is usually the most important person in your life. He or she is also the one person other than you who is most directly affected by your physical condition.

Other people, however, can behave in ways that unknowingly (on their part and possibly on yours) have a harmful influence on you. This is true even when they have the best of intentions. These behaviors fall into a few well-known patterns, described next. For the sake of understanding, we portray common behavior patterns in the most extreme manner. Most people do not fit into "type" this dramatically, but you may recognize some characteristics of each type of person in your family and friends.

Protective Family Member, Partner, or Friend

If your friend is the *protective* type, he or she may humor you as much as possible and shield you from things for which you should be responsible. They continually take everything out of your hands, believing they are protecting you. If you feel demeaned by this and suddenly get angry or even assert yourself, the protective-type friend resignedly accepts your outbursts and may then be condescending.

A protective-type friend does not bother you with his or her problems and instructs others (children, family, friends, neighbors) not to make their problems known to you. They may believe this is helpful "training," so these people will not upset you. When hearing you are in pain, these people will try to get you into bed as quickly as possible. They promptly bring you medication or call the doctor.

A protective-type friend may not like others to help you because they feel that this might be an indication of personal failure on their part. They continually say, "Let me do that." They act as if they want you to remain dependent on them. Obviously, we have painted an extreme caricature, but some of these characteristics may ring a bell.

How does your protective-type friend feel about him- or herself? Your friend feels indispensable, valuable, and good.

How do you feel when your protective-type friend practices overly solicitous behavior? You might feel that your friend mistrusts you by withholding "upsetting" information and by swooping in to help at the drop of a hat; this is not good for your self-confidence.

Pain-Denying Family Member, Partner, or Friend

A *pain-denying* type of person usually assumes that your pain cannot be as bad as you say. They cannot accept your losses in the areas of daily functioning and your feelings about these losses. They encourage you repeatedly to be strong (subtly suggesting that you are not). They often bring up other people in worse circumstances as examples. "Think about the paralyzed person who can't even get around without a wheelchair," they might say. They are also not above using themselves as an example: "I've had pain too, but I didn't let it get me down as it does you."

Especially when you want to rest during the day, they are critical. They may directly or indirectly suggest that you are giving in to the pain or, worse, that you are exaggerating and just lazy. The pain-denying person ignores your need for rest. Particularly when in the company of others, he or she may tell you not to be a wimp (or a whiner). The message is loud and clear. You should just suck it up and tough it out.

When you are feeling upset, the pain-denying person makes it clear that you should not be so emotional or weak. They often refuse to comfort you when you need it. For some people, this pattern of behavior might be due to fear: "If I validate your pain, I might make it worse," they think. It could also be due to resentment or frustration, which can even make them feel aggressive.

When you are around someone who denies your pain, you may feel guilt, shame, anxiety, or rejection, among other things. Sometimes a person will periodically swing from the protective-type to the pain-denying pattern and back again. This is even more confusing.

Indifferent Family Member, Partner, or Friend

Now let's discuss the worst type of all, the indifferent type. This type of person pays no attention to you anymore and goes his or her own way. They may be indifferent to your pain, or they may think that any efforts they make on your behalf are useless—so why bother even trying? In response, you likely feel lonely, abandoned, or depressed. You deserve better, and hopefully, you find other people who care and are willing to put forth an effort to understand.

What you need is a fourth type of significant other, a respectful type.

Respectful Family Member, Partner, or Friend

Respectful-type friends take your pain and feelings seriously. They talk with you about ways they can or cannot be of help. They don't offer more than they can do, and they assume you will arrange for other help if they're not available. They do not treat you as a patient or as someone "less than" themselves but as an equal person—someone who has pain but with whom they can still share both the good and the bad times in life. The respectful-type friend does not feel invulnerable to the kind of pain you are experiencing.

A respectful-type person understands that you will experience negative emotions as a result of your chronic pain, but they do not allow you to take it out on them. They express confidence that you can gain control and make progress in managing your pain, without minimizing the effort involved. They listen and act as a sounding board rather than attempt to solve problems for you. When they face difficulties, they ask you to listen and be a sounding board as well. They share their own vulnerabilities and limits with you.

Please note that this description is just as much of a caricature as our descriptions of protective and pain-denying people. Few people behave in a respectful manner in all ways and at all times. They have good and bad days, as well.

If you are in a family, partnership, or friendship with someone who is protective, pain-denying, or indifferent, the most you can hope for is that they will grow and change to become more respectful at least some of the time. But no one is perfect all of the time. And change, as you well know, takes time and effort.

If you have a family member, partner, or friend who is willing, you may wish to ask whether they would read this section of the book after you have made a good-faith effort to communicate more effectively. You might use it as a way to begin a dialogue about the pain problem and how it mutually affects you both. Perhaps you may only learn about their feelings. This is okay for now, as long as your partner or friend is not disrespectful. They may have kept their feelings hidden longer than you have, or they may have enacted their feelings in ways they are not proud of. You can model the patience that you hope they will have with you by accepting them where they are today.

PARTNER INTIMACY AS COMMUNICATION

Most people know the importance of warm physical contact, especially when one is not feeling well. In any circumstances, such intimacy can help you be your true self, feel appreciated, and feel safe. Unfortunately, in our society, physical contact can be threatening and may seem less natural than it really is.

Couples in which one partner experiences chronic pain often experience difficulties in the area of sexual intimacy. Sexual intercourse, for example, may be more difficult and less pleasurable as a result of pain and fatigue. Both people may unintentionally avoid physical contact. Also, people often do not have the same needs for physical intimacy at the same time. In the case of sexual intimacy, if one partner longs for tenderness and another for sexual intercourse, unless they understand this, they may reach an impasse.

Fears of failure may disturb the kind of safe atmosphere both partners need to be sexually intimate. For example, wanting to "perform well" and to give and receive orgasm can disrupt a night of romance. Outside of physical intimacy, wanting to do well in your eyes or the eyes of the other can also seriously disrupt feelings of security and intimacy with the other person. In these cases, you may feel that you are doing something *for* the other instead of *with* him or her.

It takes good communication skills to discuss intimacy and sexuality and negotiate differences in needs for physical contact. A person must feel free to say no to something and to do so in a way that does not hurt the other. This is true in other areas as well. Because pain, tiredness, stress, and uncertainty now play a role in your life, what used to be pleasurable may no longer be so. For example, pain may limit the frequency of the outings you used to go on with a best friend. He or she may not be happy with this and could even be a bit miffed. Feeling free to say no without feeling guilty, even when the other person feels frustrated and takes it personally, is quite a feat. Still, it is vitally important that everyone learns to do this because doing "yes" and thinking "no" (playacting) causes tension and may boomerang into other areas of a relationship. Ultimately, it may result in a relationship ending or getting stalled at a superficial level.

Being Romantic

Being romantic may feel like the furthest thing from your mind. But if you make your wishes known, you may find it relaxing and comforting to be in the intimate company of a person with whom you can be your true self. Being romantic does not necessarily mean being sexual, but it does go beyond friendship. Being romantic may or may not lead to sexual intimacy.

Many people find it romantic to be near a fireplace in winter, to listen to soft music, to have a favorite beverage, to share a favorite video. Others find sharing a big easy chair or comfy couch, holding hands, and watching a sunset romantic.

What is romantic to one person, however, may not be romantic to the other. One of our patients finds it romantic to wash and dry the dishes with her husband. Her husband feels like this is simply sharing a chore. However, he feels running errands together is romantic, whereas she feels it is quite stressful. They have to find a mutual ground where both feel relaxed in each other's company and in which closeness can happen naturally.

By itself, warm, safe bodily contact can have a relaxing influence. Touching tenderly, caressing, and nestling safely with each other can all bring feelings of safety and relaxation. It can be a relief (if not necessarily relaxing the first time) when two people try to openly, honestly, and confidentially explain to each other what they find relaxing and what they don't when they are together. These conversations may or may not have words. When there is respect for each other's preferences and values, when there is no shaming, and when communication is open, trust in the other person grows, and clarity and understanding result.

In any relationship, both people have to pay attention to what the other enjoys. Neither person bears responsibility for the quality of the entire relationship. Both must find the time, or make the time, to practice patience in learning to communicate and engage in further intimacy in ways that help the relationship grow.

Tips for Relationship Maintenance

Just as a car's engine will burn up if the oil is not changed and replenished, relationships need tune-ups and daily maintenance. These relationship-maintenance steps help both people act in ways that help the other and create intimacy. Here are some other steps to keep in mind:

- Remember to balance your immediate needs with the needs of the long-term relationship.

- Be gentle when you talk and when you touch.

- Try not to judge your significant other when they are not at their best. Perhaps they have reasons completely aside from the relationship for not agreeing to a request. Avoid thinking (much less saying), "If she loved me she would . . ." "If he were a good person, he would . . ." Even internal monologues of this sort can bring you down.

- Listen and be genuinely interested in the other person's point of view.

- Try not to interrupt or talk over the person.

- Use appropriate humor to help each other get over the rough spots that occur in any relationship.

While you are reading these suggestions, you might be thinking that it would be great if your significant other would read and heed them. But remember, people change more by example than they do by a lecture. And someone has to start first (usually the most motivated person in the relationship).

Also, keep in mind that troubles in a relationship take time to harden, and they take time to melt. So, don't expect dramatic changes in your communication and relationships overnight. Don't get discouraged if your first attempts do not lead to dramatic changes. Keep trying, and you will likely see some of the changes you desire.

SUMMARY

- There is a great deal of ignorance about pain and chronic pain in particular. Therefore, it may be difficult to find people who automatically understand your situation.

- By understanding where others are coming from, you can exercise effective communication skills.

- Even if no one but you changes, at the very least, you will like looking at yourself in the mirror more if you put some of these suggestions into practice. And the person who looks back at you in the mirror is the person whose opinion of you counts the most.

- The quality of communication determines whether problems cause distancing between people or whether they strengthen and deepen the bonds between them. The fact that pain is invisible, that a person with pain may outwardly look quite healthy, makes communication more difficult.

- Let people know how you feel and how you wish to be treated.

- You can identify supportive and nonsupportive behaviors in others and maximize the time you share with the supportive people while minimizing the amount of time you share with nonsupportive people.
  - Protective people humor you as much as possible, display much pity, and treat you as a patient, not a person.
  - Pain-denying people do not take you seriously; they may belittle you. They encourage you to be strong; they cannot stand when you are emotional or distressed.
  - Indifferent people are distant and avoid you. They are annoyed by your behavior and express frustration with negative comments or distance.
  - Respectful people listen to you and are responsive to your needs and wishes. They express confidence that you can come to control the pain. They take you and your pain seriously. They allow you to share your problems but do not attempt to solve all of them for you. Forming this type of relationship with someone is a process, not an outcome.
- When faced with difficult interactions, you can choose constructive ways to express or assert yourself. You can't always teach others how to be helpful, but you can reinforce helpful behaviors that others demonstrate toward you.

QUESTIONS TO CONSIDER

1. Do you feel isolated and lonely because of your pain? What does this look like for you?

2. Are there certain activities your partner or significant others do not do anymore because of your pain problem? Are there things you do not do together anymore?

3. What do you need most when you are in pain? What do you not need?

4. How do others know you are in pain? Ask your partner to see whether the messages you send are accurately understood. On the flip side, find out whether you are listening well and responding to others' concerns.

5. How do your significant others react to your pain problem? Is your partner or significant other best described as a protective type, pain-denying type, indifferent type, or a respectful type?

6. Do you think that people close to you understand how you feel and know what you want? Do you feel disappointed or encouraged by their reactions? Would your partner or significant other agree with you? Do you make clear what you want and do not want?

7. What could you tell your significant others that would be most helpful to you? How will you tell them in a way that is assertive, rather than aggressive or nonassertive?

HOME ACTIVITIES

1. The following practice exercise may help you describe your pain problem to important family members and friends who may be concerned and possibly confused about how best to help you.

   – Imagine that you are out to dinner with a significant other, and you are having a significant increase in pain. Your significant other sees the grimace on your face and asks you what is wrong. What do you say? Write the answer in your journal or notebook.

   – Identify what it is that you want from this imaginary interaction with your significant other. Do you want your significant other to listen, to offer you some reassurance, to offer you some advice, or to offer you some assistance? Would you explain your grimace any differently? In your journal or notebook, try rewriting your first sentence to include a clear request for what you may want from the interaction.

   – What kind of different response do you think that you might get after having rephrased the question to more accurately reflect what you want from the interaction?

2. Refer to the tips listed under "Improving Communication" at least once each time you anticipate interacting with other people for a week. Did you see any changes in your behavior or communication style from how you normally behave or communicate? Write down what you noticed in your notebook or journal.

3. How does your partner know that you are in pain? Ask him or her to see whether you are on the same page.

4. Arrange a time with someone important to you to discuss your thoughts, feelings, and preferences about what kind of help you want when you are in pain. It might be best to do this on one of your easier days when your pain is less severe than usual. Write down a day and time to do this.

   – Write down a second date and time in case you are not able to have this discussion, or you feel you should spend more time in this discussion.

   – How did they react to your request for a discussion? How did the conversation go? How do you feel now that you've had this discussion? Are there other things you would like to say to those close to you? If yes, write them down in your notebook or journal.

5. Think of a difficult situation that recurs in your relationship with someone. Describe the situation and then outline how you might express or assert yourself differently in the future and how you might reinforce helpful behavior on the part of the other.

PAIN SELF-ASSESSMENT, HALFWAY POINT

After you have completed this lesson, you will be more than halfway through *The Pain Survival Guide* program. This will be a good point to return to some of the ratings we included at the end of the first lesson. Please answer each of the following questions. Do not go back and look at the responses you provided after Lesson 1. Just make the ratings at this point.

Later, we suggest you go back and compare your response at different points along the program, but do not go back now. By the end of the program, we expect that you will see changes and improvements. Living with pain is a process, not an outcome. We are confident that with continued effort, you will see positive changes occurring in your life.

If you have not already done so, please photocopy this and the next page, date it, and put it in your journal or notebook. You can also download the self-assessment from http://pubs.apa.org/books/supp/turk.

1. Rate the level of your pain at the **PRESENT MOMENT**.

0   1   2   3   4   5   6

No pain   Very intense pain

2. On average, how severe has your pain been during the **PAST WEEK**?

0   1   2   3   4   5   6

Not severe   Extremely severe

3. In general, during the **PAST WEEK**, how much did your pain interfere with daily activities?

0   1   2   3   4   5   6

No interference   Extreme interference

4. During the **PAST WEEK**, how much has your pain changed the amount of satisfaction or enjoyment you get from taking part in social and recreational activities?

0   1   2   3   4   5   6

No change   Extreme change

Some of these questions can also be found on the West Haven-Yale Multidimensional Pain Inventory (Kerns, Turk, & Rudy, 1985).

5. During the **PAST WEEK**, how well do you feel that you have been able to deal with your problems?

0   1   2   3   4   5   6

Not at all   Extremely well

6. During the **PAST WEEK**, how successful were you in coping with stressful situations in your life?

0   1   2   3   4   5   6

Not successful   Extremely successful

7. During the **PAST WEEK**, how irritable have you been?

0   1   2   3   4   5   6

Not irritable   Extremely irritable

8. During the **PAST WEEK**, how tense or anxious have you been?

0   1   2   3   4   5   6

Not anxious or tense   Extremely anxious or tense

Changing Behavior

You are more likely to act yourself into feeling than to feel yourself into action.
—JEROME BRUNER

Quite naturally, people with chronic pain want to gain control over their pain and their lives. In other words, they don't want to be dependent on their pain and other people. That has been a message repeated throughout this book. But do you really know what it means to be dependent on your pain? You are dependent on (therefore, not in control of) your pain when you allow the amount and severity of your pain to determine

- what you do and how long you do it,
- whether you rest and how long you rest,
- what your mood is,
- whether you take medication and how much,
- whether you ask for help,
- whether you avoid being active or any specific activity, and
- with whom you socialize.

However, you can become more independent of your pain if you choose to change your behavior. Knowing what to change and actually doing it are two very different things, as you well know. Even the best of intentions is not enough—you have to change the way you behave. Often, what we want to do is undermined by habits about which we're not even aware. To change these patterns, we begin by helping you learn to recognize what things negatively affect your behavior and what factors are most likely to help you change. We call these the *laws of learning.*

In this lesson, we show you how your life and your pain are influenced by the attention given to certain behaviors by both yourself and others with whom you interact. Most important, we show how to change this attention pattern to increase confidence and gain independence from your pain to an extent you never dreamed possible.

REWARD DESIRABLE BEHAVIOR!

The most important law of learning is that all behavior is influenced by the consequences of the behavior—that is, the results or responses that follow from behavior—whether these consequences are self-induced or are the result of the responses of others.

Typically, if the consequences are positive, the behavior (good, desirable, or not so good or undesirable) will increase and continue. If the results are negative (undesirable, result in unwanted outcomes), the behavior will decrease or will be less likely to recur. In other words, if you do something and that action is followed by something you like (a positive reward, what you want), it is more likely that you will perform the same or similar actions in the same or similar situations. All of us hope to continue to enjoy positive or desirable outcomes.

If what you do is followed by something you do not like or want, you will be less likely to perform the same or similar action again in the same or similar circumstances. You have to learn the all-important influence of giving attention or ignoring behavior. You've probably heard the adage "the squeaky wheel always gets the grease." However, you may not be aware of how you are greasing your squeaky wheels and ignoring the ones that are quiet. That is because most automatic behaviors become less conscious over time. Also, others with whom you are in contact may, out of habit, reward those behaviors that keep you dependent on your pain and ignore those behaviors that could help you become freer to accomplish what you want. But let's begin by considering a fairly common example that has nothing to do with pain itself but illustrates these laws of learning and the effects of consequences on behavior.

Five-year-old Katy wants her mother to buy her some new boots with shockingly bright colors (neon orange and green on a black background). Her mother says no and explains that these boots are too expensive. Katy keeps asking her mother for the boots and refuses to consider any of the other less expensive pairs in the store. Her mother repeats her earlier remarks and tells Katy to select another pair (all the others are within the desired budget). Katy now starts to cry loudly and stomps her feet, making quite a scene in the store. Her mother tries to soothe and quiet her but to no avail. Katy's behavior becomes even more dramatic, and she finally throws a full-blown temper tantrum. What is a likely response from her mother?

You have likely witnessed such situations or perhaps been in them yourself, either as a child, parent, grandparent, or friend. If you were the parent, you might have given in. You were embarrassed, tired, the boots weren't *that* expensive, and someone was waiting for you. Whatever the circumstances, we have all been guilty of giving in to inappropriate behavior at some point, some of us more so than others.

The important question for our purposes here is if her mother gives in, what has Katy learned from her experience with the boots? She has begun to grasp, perhaps even without words, that if she behaves badly in front of others, she is more likely to get what she wants. That may not have been the initial intention of her tantrum (she may have been hungry and tired). But her tantrum produced the desired outcome—she obtained the boots (the reward, the outcome) she wanted.

The next time Katy wants something her mother is against, how might she act? She may begin, consciously or unconsciously, to enact in other circumstances and with other adults the same behavior that won her the boots. If she is successful in this or other attempts to have more power than a little girl should, the negative behavior will become even more deeply ingrained. Note that we are not saying Katy is a "bad girl" but that learning experiences are powerful reinforcements of behavior. The more behaviors are positively rewarded (result in the desired outcome), the more difficult they are to change. Now let's consider the complementary learning lesson—punishing desirable behavior.

Why and how would anyone try to punish, and thereby reduce the frequency of, desirable behavior? No one does this consciously. However, we do it all the time when we focus on what is inappropriate and ignore what is correct or reasonable. Another way of putting it is that we pay attention to our own or other's behaviors in a selective fashion. This is a much more difficult-to-undo learning experience, and it occurs whenever desirable behavior may be "expected" and receives no attention or no positive consequences (reinforcement). Desirable behavior is, in effect, taken for granted. In the long run, behavior that receives no attention (that is, behavior that is ignored) often disappears without anyone knowing why.

Again, let's look at a child, this time in his home environment. Six-year-old Crosby is quietly playing with his toys, and his father is quietly going about his business, either relieved that no more demands are being made of him (he has had a tough day) or perhaps simply not wishing to interfere with his son's age-appropriate play behavior. Crosby's father feels that all is going well. He does not notice Crosby looking up at him from time to time. After a while, Crosby gives up on his father, stops his creative play, and turns on the television.

Crosby's desirable behavior—namely, playing quietly—received no attention or reward from his father. In effect, he was ignored. However, we can by now guess that if he whined, he would likely get some attention, even if it was negative. For children who are feeling ignored, negative attention is better than no attention at all.

Is Crosby's father a bad parent? No, but is he behaving in a way that will increase his son's desirable behavior in the future? The answer here is no, as well.

Unfortunately, by the time we reach adulthood, we have learned from others not to be as attentive to appropriate behaviors compared with undesirable behaviors. The latter are more demanding of attention and elicit a response.

ATTENTION: A NATURAL NEED

All people need and want attention—adults as well as children—and will behave in ways to achieve it. It is human nature to attempt to see ourselves in the eyes of the ones we love and value, and if we can only see ourselves in their eyes when we practice certain negative behaviors, it is those behaviors that will become patterns in our lives. This occurs most often without conscious awareness.

As a parent, for example, you try to be consistent. You systematically try to reward good behavior and punish bad behavior, either directly by your response or by ignoring it. But does that happen as often as you would like? In the examples of the children Katy and Crosby, you can observe the laws of learning in action. In both cases, providing a reward—orange boots or attention—will likely increase the child's behavior in new situations. In Crosby's case, consistent failure to provide acknowledgment or praise for desirable behavior will likely lead to a reduction in appropriate behavior. In these ways, reinforcement can lead to an increase in negative behavior and a decrease in positive behavior.

Let's see how this works with adults by considering Sandra and Scott, a married couple. Scott likes reading his newspaper and watching TV every night. He only half listens to his wife as she tries to tell him about her day. Without meaning to, his behavior is telling her that what she has to say is less interesting and important than the TV or newspaper. When Sandra asks him to pay attention to her, he either ignores her or behaves as if she is being childish and demanding.

Sandra may respond to Scott's behavior in several ways. She may grumble under her breath, she may get outwardly angry, or she may unconsciously forget to pass on an important message one of Scott's friends told her yesterday. She may not be aware of any of these responses, or she may be aware of some. This is an important point: Behavioral responses can occur without conscious intention or even awareness. They may become automatic.

Assume that none of Sandra's efforts are successful, and Scott continues to be unresponsive to her best efforts to gain his attention. In desperation, and to be overly dramatic, Sandra announces that she wants a divorce and begins packing her bags. Suddenly, she has Scott's attention.

Scott does not want a divorce. He changes immediately, and suddenly he is ready to give Sandra his undivided attention. He promises to read less and pay more attention to Sandra, and he brings her flowers the next day.

What has Sandra learned from this experience? She observes that only when she takes extreme measures (not quite tantrums, as in the example of Katy, though the result is the same) will Scott respond in the way she wishes. Packing her bags was followed by the desired outcome (Scott's undivided attention and changed behavior). Remember, behavior that produces a desirable outcome will be repeated—a basic law of learning. What do you think Sandra will be likely to do the next time Scott is inattentive?

Let's consider another example. José hurt his back on the job several years ago. His severe pain has affected all parts of his life. He mostly sits in his lounge chair watching TV during the day and stays in bed watching TV at night. He visited a physical therapist who developed an exercise plan for him, making use of the principles of pacing we described in Lesson 2. But every time José tried the exercises, he felt that his pain became worse, and he feared that the exercises would cause more serious damage to his back. So, whenever he started to be active, he used the first sign of pain to stop his exercise and lie down. When he did, his pain seemed somewhat reduced (stopping exercise achieved a positive outcome: less pain).

This example shows how we can produce what we think are "desirable outcomes" by ourselves. What has Jose learned from his experience? Several things: "If it hurts, don't do it"; "Exercise causes pain, so don't do exercise"; and "If I stop exercising and lie down, my pain is relieved. So, stop at any sign of pain to achieve the desired outcome."

José has also come to connect activity with pain. Now, even if physical therapy is mentioned, he may feel his back start to act up. It is like the famous dog that Pavlov taught to salivate at the sound of a bell because that sound was previously associated with getting fed. Pavlov's dog had learned to anticipate and expect food when he heard a bell. When the bell sounded, food followed, and the dog, in anticipation of the food, began to salivate. Over time, when the bell went off, even when no food was present, the dog began to salivate. The dog, like José, learned to expect something to happen on the basis of previous learning and behaved accordingly.

What impact do you think José's experience will have on his general behavior? As you might expect, he will become more and more inactive in anticipation of the undesirable consequences (namely, increased pain). The more inactive he is, the more he loses muscle strength, flexibility, and endurance. Thus, another vicious circle is created, and physical limitations increase and more activities become difficult and painful.

Learning to avoid something, like activity, to prevent an undesired outcome is referred to as *avoidance learning*. It is a variant of the first law of learning (that all behavior is influenced by the consequences of that behavior). In the case of chronic pain, learning to anticipate undesired outcomes (for example, pain) will cause one to avoid healthy behavior such as staying active.

TABLE 6.1. Consequences of Behavior Examples

Behavior	Consequence	Reinforcement	Result
Katy throwing tantrum	Giving in	Positive	More tantrums
Crosby quietly playing	No attention, neglect	No reinforcement	No longer playing
Sandra asking for attention	No attention, neglect	No reinforcement	No longer asking
Sandra packing her bags	Much attention, flowers every Friday	Positive reinforcement	More attention seeking, flowers become predictable and ignored
José exercising	More pain and worry	Negative	No more exercising
José lying down	Less pain and worry	Positive	More resting

Table 6.1 summarizes behavior based on both laws of learning presented in this lesson in case examples. Rewards are considered positive reinforcement, whereas undesired outcomes are considered punishment.

THE LAWS OF LEARNING AND YOU

How does attention work in day-to-day relationships? On the positive side, when we look for good behavior in others and give attention to these positive elements in our relationships, these relationships will steadily become stronger and closer. That's what tends to happen when one rewards the positive behaviors in relationships by giving them more attention.

However, if we are continually busy discovering faults in others (our partner, colleagues, boss, or children), and if we criticize or attack others frequently, we punish their experience of being around us. Likewise, if we ignore their support and efforts to be helpful, their positive behaviors will decrease, and they may become angry or withdraw their efforts, as we noted in the case of Janet's husband and children in Lesson 5.

For some people, complaints of pain get more and more attention, and this attention influences their behavior in a negative way. For others, feeling pain and maintaining a positive disposition may well be ignored—remember how the squeaky wheel gets the grease. Therefore, people who didn't complain at first about their pain may begin to talk about it or show more and more nonverbal signs of suffering to obtain a desired response, such as attention.

Negative attention may be unpleasant, but when we receive no attention, we feel as if we might disappear. That's why it's natural, although counterproductive, for an adult to seek attention through talking and complaining about pain. The key is to try to find ways to receive needed attention when it is desired without reinforcing one's sense of suffering and perhaps driving others away.

TABLE 6.2. Summary of the Laws of Behavior Learning

Action	Consequences	Probability of the behavior recurring
Positive reinforcement	Reward the behavior	More likely
Negative reinforcement	Prevent or withdraw, avoid	More likely
Punishment	Negative responses and much attention	More likely
Punishment	Ignoring the behavior, little attention	Less likely
Neglect	Prevent or withdraw positive results	Less likely

By way of review, we have summarized the behavioral principles behind the laws of learning in Table 6.2.

WHAT ARE THE CONSEQUENCES OF MISPLACING YOUR ATTENTION?

We have seen that attention has a strong power to influence behavior. But specifically, what kinds of attention are desirable and undesirable when it comes to chronic pain? Is it good to give your pain as much attention as possible, or is it better to ignore it? You may be surprised by the answers.

Health Care Provider Shopping

We have talked about the role of responses to behavior and used the examples of children, marital couples, and someone with chronic pain. But the role of responses to behavior applies to health care providers as well. Doctors and other health care providers often unwittingly reinforce pain by paying particular attention to increased reporting of pain. The more pain reported, the more attention they give the patient. The opposite is also true. When people report a reduction of pain, they often receive less attention from their health care provider. This may have unfortunate results.

Let's consider how health care providers may influence patients' behaviors. If a patient goes to a physician who has prescribed pain medication and says his pain is no better, and the physician increases the dose with the effect of a small reduction in pain, what will the patient learn? Complaining of pain led to increased medication and some pain reduction. If pain is reduced, even a little, the next time the patient reports to his physician that his pain is better, the physician may think things are getting better and not increase the dose. However, if the patient says he still has a lot of pain despite the increased dose, and the report is followed by the physician prescribing an even greater dose increase or a more potent drug, the patient has learned that complaining led to increased attention and more medication (similar to Katy and the boots), whereas saying the pain was reduced resulted in no increased medication, and pain persists.

So, complaining had a positive effect, whereas not complaining lead to no positive reinforcement (not even a small additional pain reduction). The same thing would occur if the patient informed his physical therapist that the exercises prescribed increased the pain. Here the physical therapist might reduce the exercises recommended. In both instances, complaining lead to a reinforcement—more pain medication, less demanding exercises—whereas not complaining did not produce any desirable outcome. So, in these instances, what will the patient likely learn and do?

When a health care provider no longer provides attention, patients may begin to think about repeating diagnostic tests or searching out new therapies or health care providers. Placing one's hopes on a health care provider or treatment is natural in the beginning. It decreases feelings of aloneness and engenders hope—at least something is being tried to bring relief. However, although new health care providers or new treatments may generate hope at first, they may then lead to deeper feelings of hopelessness, distress, and a frantic search for other options as relief of pain is not achieved. Continual health care shopping will eventually bring about increasingly more despair because false hopes and attention will not in themselves reduce pain.

However, some people with chronic pain stay with the same health care provider, but they become dependent on him or her for too long a time. This results in a fearful dependence and uncertainty, often followed by a lack of hope, frustration, and distress. If the distress brings about attention at that point, they may receive a lot of punishment for emphasizing their pain.

Only the right kind of attention can take one's mind off the pain and focus it toward more productive areas. What does this look like in practice? It may be that the health care provider invites the patient to come in on a regular basis and not only when the pain is most severe. He or she gives the patient attention on good days, not just bad ones, explains that drugs are not the only solution, and acknowledges the patient's efforts to self-manage the pain.

Think about your experiences. How many specialists have you sought out? How many medications and treatments have you tried? How many surgeries have you received? How did you feel when a new treatment was recommended? If your hopes for the new treatment were dashed, how did you feel?

Endless searching for "something new" will also interfere with your attempts to self-manage your pain. Many products and treatments hold out promises of relief. But do their sponsors have any real evidence to back up their claims, and are these claims appropriate for someone like you? We're not talking about personal testimonials or media advertisements but clear scientific proof—not nine out of 10 doctors or assertions that "many patients achieve wonderful outcomes" but real scientific data. The energy you spend seeking unproven treatments or the next new "miracle" takes time away from learning proven methods that help reduce both pain and distress and that lead you to a better life.

At some point, all of us must accept ownership of our lives. If you have gotten this far in the book, you have begun this journey toward resilience and reclaiming your life. Over time, you will see the benefits in your ability to do more and enjoy activities and in improvements in your relationships with other people.

Trying to Fool All the People All the Time—and Failing

Some people try to hide their pain. They think that hiding the pain causes less distress to those around them. After all, putting on a false happy face may reduce unwanted questions and undesired attention. Too much attention may become annoying and painful in itself.

However, hiding your pain all the time is not a good idea. Denying a part of reality (the pain) means that you continually have to play a false role; you continually have to walk on eggshells—in short, you can never be yourself. Covering up takes a lot of energy. Trying to fool all the people all the time is exhausting. And it is impossible to fool yourself.

But wait a minute, you might say! Wasn't the first part of this lesson devoted to the hidden costs of bringing others' attention to your pain? Yes, that is true. That is where our emphasis was. But you may remember that we also discussed the benefits of sharing, engaging in open and honest communication, and obtaining and giving the right kind and amount of attention (see Lesson 5).

First, you need some attention with regard to your distress. Without someone validating your pain or by not allowing yourself to receive appropriate attention, you may be spending more of your attention on your pain. This then magnifies your experience of pain.

To receive this validation, you have to be honestly open about your pain and limitations with appropriate people at appropriate times. That is, you need to let the *right someone* in on what you are truly experiencing, someone with whom you can be your real self. If you have no one in your life at this time who fits that bill, share your feelings with God, a higher power, or even the "benign universe."

Accentuating the Negative

As we discussed before, the squeaky wheels in our lives get the grease, not only from others but also, more important, from ourselves. This is partly because when things are going well, we quickly consider the positive to be normal and give it little attention. Anything outside of this automatically receives our attention.

Think back to the last time you had a bad cold. For a few days after the cold had passed, you felt grateful for the fact that you could breathe normally, that your nose wasn't raw, and that your nose and sinuses did not feel congested. You felt grateful to be able to do all the normal things that you usually took for granted. After a while, however, you forgot what it was like to have a cold, and breathing easily felt normal again.

Chronic pain, by its very nature, does not go away like a cold. So, it is easy to get stuck on focusing on the negative—the pain. This naturally leads to negative thoughts and emotions. We are not telling you to deny your pain. What we are saying is that if you give it more attention than it is due, you end up paying a double price for it. You not only have the pain you started with, but now you also have more negative emotions, more negative thoughts, and an intensified experience of pain.

Think for a moment about all the distressing emotions humans can feel: anger, fear, depression, shame, guilt, jealousy, sadness, embarrassment, and annoyance, to name just a few. Now, think of all the pleasurable emotions humans can feel. Were you able to come up with as many? Most people, when asked to think about it, can name more negative emotions than positive ones (for example, happiness, contentment, success, optimism). It takes work to focus on positive emotions (we return to this in Lesson 7).

Think again about your health and body. When they were functioning properly, you may have hardly given it a thought. Most healthy people do not pay much attention to their bodies unless they are trying to lose weight or are temporarily ill.

Acknowledge to yourself not only when you are in pain but also when you have a good day or even when you feel just a bit better in one part of your body. Try to appreciate this and whatever other positive emotions you may feel. On good days (and on bad days), try focusing on what you can do or what you have, such as moving more easily or having a varied daily schedule. Try to focus on the small things—a smile from the mail carrier or a phone call from a friend.

And don't be afraid to admit to yourself when you feel better, physically or emotionally. It will not "jinx" your improvement. It won't give you false hope unless you tell yourself, "Now, I'm well for good." This is not realistic. As in most things, it's best to take one day at a time.

On difficult days, you may want to focus more on the parts of your body that function well, quietly stimulating and activating them. This can start a cycle of feeling a bit better, leading to more pleasant emotions and positive behaviors and feeling even better. On any day, easy or challenging, you can focus on the healthy parts of your body and what you can do or look forward to doing. Perhaps using the relaxation exercises described in Lesson 3 can help you strengthen this focus.

The well-functioning areas of your body deserve as much of your attention as your pain. We give more attention to the role of your thoughts and how to modify these when appropriate in the next lesson, Lesson 7.

HOW EXACTLY DO REWARDS FOR BEHAVIOR WORK?

You now know that when you pay attention to positive (healthy, well) behavior, that act is already a positive step. What's important next is to recognize how you can use your attention effectively as a reward to achieve positive results for yourself and others.

Four factors determine the effectiveness of any reward or reinforcement: *desirability* (how positive the reward is to you or another person), *timing* (how close the reward is to the behavior that is to be reinforced), *frequency* (how often), and *predictability*. The reward is most effective if it is

- something that is desired by you or someone else,
- provided as soon as possible after the desirable behavior,
- given frequently, and
- timed in an unpredictable way.

Desired Rewards

Whatever the reward is, it must be viewed favorably by the person to whom it is directed. For example, if you gave someone a box of candy as a reward, and they were eating a low sugar diet to control diabetes, the reward might not be desired. In the case of pain, someone who tells you to take it easy because you do not "look good today" might not be rewarding you if you are trying to do more to build up your endurance. To be positive, the reward, whether attention or some tangible object, has to be something the recipient wishes to receive. The more desirable it is, the more reinforcing and motivating it is.

Prompt Rewards

Rewards are most effective if they follow the behavior to be reinforced closely in time. To illustrate what this means, we use an example about alcohol and the potential person with alcoholism.

Someone taking his or her first drink often experiences a reduction in anxiety and worry and an increase in relaxation and sociability as a result of the alcohol. Drinking is thus immediately positively rewarded by these desirable feelings. In fact, anticipating these positive feelings may lead to taking the next drink and drinking the next day and the day after that. If a person becomes an alcoholic, he or she may experience many negative consequences later on (for example, loss of job, family, prestige). However, it's clear why people with alcoholism find it hard to quit, when you consider that the initial feeling of pleasure or anticipation of pleasure that is reinforced soon after a drink may be much more influential than these negative consequences at a later date.

When people with alcoholism are sober, they may be aware of the losses involved with drinking and may feel miserable, guilty, and ashamed. Also, when sober, the person with alcoholism may experience people and situations in his or her environment as punishing, therefore punishing the state of being sober. However, as soon as he or she takes a drink, these undesirable emotions and punishments seem to fade away. Problems are soon forgotten, and only the present state of relief counts—not yesterday and certainly not tomorrow.

The same can be true for chronic pain. You may feel relatively worthless one day because you have done so little, according to your standards. Then, you feel somewhat better the next day, so you overdo it to make up for the perceived lack of accomplishment yesterday. During the activity, you may feel fairly well. You taste the satisfaction of being occupied, there is a diversion, and there is often a visible result. You feel somewhat better about yourself. So, what's the catch?

The catch is that you are not punished immediately for doing too much or for doing it too long. The pain typically comes later—the next day or the day after that. It is only then that you discover you have gone beyond your limitations (think pacing!). The link between behavior and punishment is too far apart in time to be helpful.

Progressing too fast in your activity plan or staying active until you are in pain and are fatigued will feel like a delayed sunburn after enjoying the sun. Or it can be subtler: If you stop your activities and rest after a certain amount of pain, rest will be the inadvertent reward that follows the pain. Strangely enough, this will cause that pain level to occur earlier and more often. This is because something good only happens when you feel the pain is extreme— namely, the body receives rest or medication. Thus, a paradox or puzzle arises. If prescription painkillers are used, they can be a positive reward for experiencing pain.

Along the same lines, perhaps you are only able to ask for attention and help when you feel the pain forces you to do so. In this manner, you will become steadily more dependent on severe pain to give you the opportunity to ask for help or get needed attention.

Maybe you think, "I'm a real fighter. I don't complain, and I don't give up quickly. I continue until I can't go on anymore. I only stop if the pain and tiredness force me to. I only take medicines when I really can't stand the pain and need them."

The flaw in this approach is that if you only rest and take drugs when you absolutely need to, you are setting yourself up for failure. Like the person with alcoholism who only drinks when he or she "needs to," you may be striding straight toward dependence on pain to bring you needed relief.

So, if your doctor has prescribed pain medication, and you have pain most of the time, it is usually best to take it at regular times each day rather than when your pain is worst. If you take pain medication only when your pain is at its worst, you inadvertently reinforce that medication is a positive reward for pain. This may actually increase the amount of pain you feel! If, however, you have episodes of pain and do not have pain all the time, or most of the time, taking your medication when you have a flare-up may be appropriate.

In summary, pain medication, rest, and attention should not be directly linked to a certain amount of pain but rather to your planned schedule. You should get rest, attention, and help even when your pain is less severe to maintain any reductions in pain. If you experience flare-ups in your pain, you might want to alter your schedule, but once the pain does lessen, you should go back to your planned activities as soon as possible. We discuss dealing with flare-ups in detail in Lesson 9.

Frequent Rewards

Small rewards given frequently tend to work better than a large reward promised in the distant future. This is especially true when a new behavior is being developed. For example, parents sometimes promise their child at the beginning of the new school year that they will buy them a much-desired bicycle or computer game if they get all *As* or high marks at the end of the semester. The parents are usually surprised to see that for most children, this incentive has little to no influence at all on daily study behavior. Smaller but more frequent rewards tend to be more motivating for consistent study behavior—for example, going to the movies or receiving a small amount of money or a small toy at the end of the week. Then, the reward will be closer in time, more frequent, and more linked to the efforts made during the week.

You, too, can only move forward by gradual but persistent effort and a willingness to stick with your self-management plan. Give yourself special attention or rewards for your efforts frequently, even when you don't see objective evidence of "success." In the same vein, try not to dwell too long on inevitable setbacks. Setbacks are to be expected. Most successful nonsmokers try at least three times before they succeed in quitting smoking for good. Remember, you learned to walk and ride a bike only by falling and getting up again.

In short, you can have long-term goals, but progress will come more quickly if you strive toward limited goals over the short term and reinforce effort and small successes along the way to longer term goals. However, make sure your goals are realistic, as we discussed in Lesson 2. Another way to tell whether your goals are realistic is the extent to which they are SMART—that is,

- **S**pecific,
- **M**easurable,
- **A**chievable or **A**ttainable,
- **R**elevant (personally meaningful) or **R**ealistic, and
- **T**imely.

It also helps if your partner and other significant people in your life understand your self-management plan and provide encouragement and positive support for your efforts and even small accomplishments. It would probably also be best if they paid little attention to any setbacks that naturally occur. We emphasize this because, too often, our patients become critical of themselves when they have not achieved their long-term goals as soon as they thought they would.

Keeping the kind of progress charts we described in Lesson 2 can provide you with immediate feedback on your efforts. Over time, you can see where you started and where you are now. For example, you can see that you started by being able to walk for 5 minutes, and now you can walk 12 minutes. This is success! Perhaps you used to be active around the house for 10-minute intervals three times a day, and now you are active for 20 minutes three times a day. This is success! Most important, however, is that you will see how you have been active in taking charge of your pain and your life.

Unpredictable Rewards

Probably the most surprising thing you will read in this lesson is that rewards are most effective when they are not predictable. If every time you played solitaire, you won, you'd be positively reinforced each time, but you would probably not find the game as interesting, and you might stop playing. Regular gamblers get "hooked" because they are rewarded in an unpredictable manner ("One more try on this slot machine, and I'll win"). One factor that may account for the appeal of fishing is that you do not know exactly when or if you are going to catch a fish. Unexpected gifts tend to be more appreciated than predictable presents on fixed dates. This is also true in a relationship. One couple we know gives each other unexpected presents throughout the year instead of on birthdays and at Christmas. They then enjoy birthdays and holidays without the added tension of gift-giving that sometimes surrounds these occasions.

Remember the example of Sandra and Scott earlier in this lesson? What we did not mention is that after learning that Sandra needed positive attention, Scott started to bring her flowers every Friday. At first, Sandra was delighted. Over time, however, bringing flowers on Friday became routine. Sandra would even forget to notice that Scott had brought flowers home. The predictability of the reward had led to it being less rewarding. Anyone who's been in a relationship knows that if Scott stopped bringing Sandra flowers, she would likely be hurt. Perhaps a fight would ensue. At the very least, Scott might hear, in an obvious or subtle accusatory voice, "Why didn't you bring any flowers?"

Thus, failure to do what comes to be expected often creates problems in a relationship. However, a certain amount of unpredictability is desirable, not only in our daily lives but also in our relationships. A certain amount of predictability provides comfort and order. But progress and other good things in life need surprise rewards; otherwise, they tend to disappear.

If you have raised children, you may have learned (or are learning) that unpredictably rewarding *undesirable* behavior makes this behavior the most stubborn and difficult to change. If a child misbehaves and sometimes you give him or her a time-out and sometimes you don't, the misbehavior is likely to continue and increase in frequency. The unpredictable nature of pain often causes people with chronic pain to gamble with their activity and rest routines. They may even rely on "Lady Luck." One day they feel well, so they think they are lucky and do a lot. A day or two later, they feel bad and rest all day, thinking, "Tomorrow, I may be lucky again." In the world of pain, however, gambling in this way only leads to loss.

PREPARING FOR BEHAVIORAL CHANGE

As people with chronic pain begin to consider behavioral changes, one problem they often face is that some of their previous behaviors were rewarding in the short term. That is, passivity, avoidance behavior, taking sleeping pills, and so on provided immediate rewards, so it was easy to become hooked on these illusory charms.

The second problem you may face as you begin to change your behavior is that you may feel punished almost immediately. Everyone feels a degree of discomfort or distress when he or she first begins to change, whether this is activity–rest cycles, relationship changes, or smoking or dietary changes. You will likely feel this, too, at first. We ask that you persevere *consistently* for at least 6 weeks. Research has shown that it takes consistent change for 6 weeks before people (a) see progress and (b) feel natural with regard to the change.

Our patients have taught us that the distress or discomfort felt at the beginning of change is heavily outweighed by the rewards of consistency over time. They also have told us that they could tolerate a lot of discomfort at first when they believed it would ultimately lead to less pain, less frequency of pain, and more enjoyment of life. Chronic pain is generally purposeless and makes people feel hopeless because it serves no purpose. If you learn to accept and to manage your pain in the ways we have described, you will make goals for yourself (SMART goals), and you will have a means of reaching that goal, one day and one step at a time. One of our patients summed this up nicely: "I used to feel controlled by my pain, but now I feel I'm in charge of my life, even though I still experience some pain!" This person overcame her fears, her felt lack of control, and her hopelessness. You can, too!

SUMMARY

- Dependence on pain occurs when pain is the driver, and you are in the back seat. You can get in the front seat and put pain in its proper place (the back seat and eventually the trunk).

- If you want to change, good motivation and willpower are not enough. It is important for you to learn and make use of the laws of learning. These laws can maintain inappropriate behavior (passivity, giving-up, dependence on medication and other treatments) and can also lead to more appropriate behavior (enhancing self-control and self-respect).

- Use rewards to increase your wellness behavior (sharing, planning, activities, scheduling rest and medications). Reward yourself when you avoid temptations such as overdoing and under-doing it, irritability, moaning, and passivity. Change from being passive, reactive, and helpless in the face of your pain to being active, resourceful, and in control!

- Effective rewards are desirable, immediate, frequent, and unpredictable.

- If you're paying the right amount of attention to your pain, you are facing reality—focusing behavior on doing what is achievable and not on what others want or expect and cherishing those moments when the body functions better and hurts less.

- Positive changes happen only by a gradual process of development. This means you will fall and get up again. Pay little attention to falling and give yourself lots of respect for getting back up again. Recording and monitoring your progress and effort, even small steps, can be an effective self-reward system.

- Most of us naturally prefer predictability in our daily routines and our relationships. The unpredictable nature of pain, however, can cause you to gamble. When you fail to pace yourself and hope you will be lucky, ignoring the pain and the real situation, this gambling will only lead to loss.

- Important changes do not always result in immediate success, but they are an investment in your future.

QUESTIONS TO CONSIDER

1. Problems increase when they get too much attention. Do you agree with this? Why or why not?

2. What are some ways you can you stop the cycle of health care provider and treatment shopping?

3. What do you value most about your partner, children, family, neighbors, friends? How do you show your appreciation?

4. What rewards are desirable, immediate, frequent, and unpredictable for you?

5. Chronic pain is unpredictable. What does this mean for you? In what ways might chronic pain be in the "driver's seat" for you? How can you kick it into the back seat or trunk?

6. Are there any activities you have learned to avoid to prevent pain? Have you noticed that, over time, there may be a greater number of activities that you avoid for fear that they will make your pain worse?

HOME ACTIVITIES

1. Take a few moments to think about what you consider important. Where would you like to devote more attention, and where would you like less emphasis—social contacts (friends, family), activities (hobby, work, study), health (condition, weight), family (partner, children)? Write down one or more SMART goals for the areas where you would like more emphasis.

2. List at least three things you can do for yourself that you would find rewarding. Use these when you achieve your SMART goals.

3. Over a couple of days, notice only your positive behaviors; pay attention to them and dwell on them. Ignore negative behaviors as much as possible.

How does this feel? If you wish, keep a reward journal for your efforts for the next 2 weeks. Record your positive behavior (for example, effort, action), how you rewarded yourself, and how you felt after the reward.

4. Over a day or two, keep track of the number of complimentary and critical statements you make to people who are important to you. Do the results surprise you and perhaps indicate a need for change on your part?

5. Every day for the next week, try to give at least one person a sincere compliment.

   Notice how they react. Notice how you feel afterward.

6. Pay attention to how people respond to you when you tell them you are having a good day or are feeling somewhat less pain.

   – Do they ignore you?
   – Do they immediately give you more responsibilities or unrewarding tasks to do?
   – Do they seem less willing to spend time with you because you appear "better"? Are they glad that they can go their own way again?
   – How does this contrast with how they respond when you tell them you are having a bad day or things are not going well?
   – Do they give you more attention?
   – Do they spend more time with you?
   – Do they get frustrated or angry?
   – If they give you less attention when you are well and feeling good, does this sometimes lead you to try to convince them of the severity of your pain? Can you see a vicious circle here?

Changing Thoughts and Feelings

Man can alter his life by altering his thinking.

—WILLIAM JAMES

Thinking is the way you talk to yourself (*self-talk*). *Feeling* is the way your emotions react to your thoughts or behavior. Thinking and feeling are very different than doing, of course. The way you think and behave influences what you feel and how much you feel.

Perhaps you are thinking at this point, "I set SMART (specific, measurable, achievable or attainable, relevant (personally meaningful) or realistic, timely) goals, and I am practicing the principles of pacing, balance, and learning. I know what I must do to succeed. How come I don't feel all that much better yet? In fact, today, I feel lousy."

Although natural, this kind of self-talk can discourage you, undermine your efforts, diminish your motivation, and lead to setbacks in your progress. Thoughts and feelings play a central role in your continuing to change, experiencing satisfaction with change, and being willing to continue working toward your goals in the face of inevitable setbacks.

In this lesson, you will learn methods that will enable you to become more aware of and influence your thoughts and feelings and, thereby, your pain. These include methods that will help you think more realistically and prevent your feelings from dictating your behavior.

METHOD 1: THINKING DIFFERENTLY

Try to recall a serious conflict you have had with someone. What feelings or emotions can you recall before, during, and after this conflict? Did you feel anger, frustration, sadness, or worry? Most likely, you were not aware of your thoughts at the time the conflict was taking place.

We would like you to consider that *how you thought* about this conflict influenced your feelings. And we would also like you to consider that these feelings then influenced the way you later thought and then how you felt—in yet another vicious circle, like the others we keep noting.

One major way our usual manner of thinking gets in our way is that our "interpretation" of problems changes the way we view and experience them. This distortion leads to feelings that are distressing. And these distressing emotions produce major negative physical changes in our bodies (for example, increase arousal, muscle tension, heart rate) and, therefore, in our experience of pain.

Our feelings also influence how we think. If we feel upset, we may think, "I didn't handle that well. I'm not good at dealing with conflicts" or "He is being really mean. I should never have married him."

A second way that distressing feelings are intensified is that we think about the conflict or our feelings too much and from only one (typically our own) perspective. This may lead to actions we regret and the negative emotions that follow those actions. We may lash out. Or we may get stuck in feeling sorry for ourselves.

Think of when you had a conflict with someone, something that got your mind and emotions all riled up. Then, unexpectedly, something else important and engaging came up, and you were distracted for a day or two. During that period, you probably did not have time to think about the conflict that was so much on your mind before. The first time you again revisited the conflict, you probably felt much less distressed. However, if you then continued to dwell on it, you likely aroused the feelings that were put aside. You actually thought yourself into the same spot you were in before you were distracted.

Thoughts and feelings are powerful. They can cause distress and affect your body and behavior, but they also can be used to help you. For example, just as it is possible to arouse negative thinking and distressing emotions, it is also possible to positively influence thinking and feeling. Although these thoughts are at times automatic, you can, at least to some extent, learn to exert control of what you think and how you feel.

In this regard, one of the real differences between a pessimist and an optimist is that the optimist focuses thoughts and feelings on positive things, whereas the pessimist focuses on the things that can and do go wrong. For someone thinking pessimistically, even the most positive situation can be viewed negatively.

In a rather exaggerated example, imagine a pleasant scene in which a couple is having a picnic on a lovely spring afternoon. They are sitting under a tree next to a small brook. In this instance, the wife sees only the positive characteristics of this scene, whereas the husband sees something quite different. She thinks about the beautiful blue sky, the shade the tree is providing, and the delicious meal to come. He, however, is thinking about the possibility that the grass might stain their clothes, that the food might get infested with ants, and that the clouds in the distance portend a storm. As he thinks about these things, he begins to believe that the storm he has conjured up may involve lightning, and they are sitting under a tree that could be struck by lightning and injure them. He begins looking at his watch to see whether they have enough time to eat before the storm arrives. Who do you think is enjoying their time more—the wife or husband?

Perhaps you are thinking, "That's all well and good for a picnic, but what about my pain? That's no picnic at all." That is true, but on a given day, how you think about your pain will influence how you think about other things that day, what emotions you experience, how you behave, your physical responses, and as a result, even how much pain you will experience.

For example, consider Melissa, who wakes up in pain and begins thinking about how hopeless her situation is, how helpless she feels to influence the pain, and how her friends are off doing things she cannot. As a result of these thoughts, she is likely feeling sad, depressed, envious, angry, or some combination of these emotions. These feelings, in turn, will increase tension in her body and create a sense of exhaustion, and both of these will add to her pain and her experience of the intensity of her pain. Remember, feelings can open the pain gate, described in Lesson 1, and make pain feel even more intense.

Common Thinking Errors

Negative and distressing thoughts also have the effect of increasing distressing feelings because they lead to focusing on the "worst possibility" in the future (your whole house is falling down). This soon grows to a probability, and you are likely to end up feeling like a helpless and hopeless captive of your pain forever. These thoughts go around and around, taking all your attention and causing your body to go into "fight-or-flight" mode (anger, tension) or into complete passivity (depression). Either way, you lose, and like Melissa, your pain increases. Pain seems to be a cruel judge, and you will soon feel as if you have a life sentence without the possibility of parole.

Fortunately, researchers and therapists have identified several patterns or categories that our negative thoughts often fall into. Why is this a good thing? Because understanding the patterns can help you recognize when you are having thoughts that might result in increased stress, tension, and pain. And if you recognize and "label" your thoughts as unhelpful, you then have the power to change them.

The following list contains some of the more common thinking errors.

- Blaming. You make someone or something else responsible for your pain: "My lousy boss caused my job accident" or "My family demands so much from me. That's why I can't afford the time or money to take care of this pain." Or the blame is turned inward: "It's all my fault that this happened to me" or "If only I hadn't . . ."

- "Should," "must," or "ought" statements. The words *should, must,* or *ought* appear regularly in negative thinking and irrational thoughts about pain. Shoulds are secret put-downs, implying that a person is stupid, foolish, or weak: "I should have thought of good body mechanics before I lifted that box"; "I shouldn't have been in such a hurry; that's why I slipped on the ice"; "I must keep up with all my responsibilities, pain or no pain"; "I shouldn't react to pain like this"; "I should know better."

- Polarized thinking. Everything is black or white, good or bad when we think in a polarized way. There is no gray area in which reality or improvement can be seen. Polarized thinking is often couched in terms of absolute statements with certain cue words such as *all, every, none, never, always, everybody,* and *nobody*: "I stopped doing my activities for 2 days, and now I'm really in pain. I'll never be able to manage my pain"; "I feel worse today than I did yesterday. My pain is never going to go away"; "I always start a program, but then I always quit. Every time is going to be the same, so what's the use?" "Everybody else can do this program. I'm always the one who can't do things"; "Nobody can help me"; "Nobody suffers as much as me."

- Catastrophizing. When we catastrophize, we react to situations by imagining the worst possible scenario or outcome: "I know that the only thing left is to have surgery. I'm sure I'll be laid up for months. Then I'll probably be worse than before." "What if" statements are often catastrophizing in disguise: "What if the operation is a failure?" "What if my pain never gets better, and I have to live like an invalid for the rest of my life?" "What if my spouse leaves me?" "What if I am unable to ever work again?"

- Control fallacies. This involves feeling or thinking that one is "externally controlled" by others, such as those in the medical profession, or that one is more in control of the outcomes of problems than one really is: "This new doctor is really going to help me. I know she's the only one"; "If I don't do it, no one will"; "Everyone depends on me. I've got to recover quickly, or the family will fall apart."

- Emotional reasoning. This line of thinking assumes that what you feel emotionally *must* be true in reality: "I'm taking too long to heal. I must be doing something wrong"; "The pain is back again full force. It's never going to stop"; "I'm useless. I'll never be able to _____ (fill in the blank) again."

- Filtering. Filtering involves seeing situations through a kind of tunnel vision. Most often, people filter out any potentially positive aspects of their lives: "This is not living. What's the use?" (ignoring the sunny day, the phone call from his son, and the delicious breakfast a neighbor fixed).

- Entitlement fallacy. Some level of pain and discomfort is a normal part of life, as are illness, loss, aging, and eventually death. Some people feel that they are "entitled" to escape these human experiences (witness the rise in cosmetic surgery): "This kind of pain isn't fair"; "Why do I have to go through this?" "My sister is older than I am, and she never experiences any pain. Why am I always the victim?"

- Overgeneralizing. This type of thinking is similar to catastrophizing. Most often, it consists of assuming that the occurrence of a single event or situation is characteristic of most, if not all, others: "I tried twice to use controlled breathing, and I don't feel any better; it's never going to work"; "If today is bad, tomorrow is surely going to be even worse."

- Mind reading. This involves making assumptions about the thoughts behind another person's words or actions: "My family avoids talking to me about my pain; they don't really care about me"; "If she really cared, she'd be here rather than out with her friends for lunch."

Examples of Choosing to Think Differently

You may think, "I'm a realist, not a pessimist." But there is a difference between "negative" thinking and "realistic thinking." In Exhibit 7.1, we list some of the negative thoughts our patients have admitted to having. Do any of them sound familiar? After working on the lessons outlined in this book, these same people learned to think more realistically. Exhibit 7.2 lists their thoughts later on. Note that the statements do not indicate that the person's pain is totally gone. Some of them indicate that a person with chronic pain is having a particularly bad pain day. But realistic thoughts have a much more positive influence on the experience of pain than negative or pessimistic thoughts, which open the pain gate.

In another example, let's imagine that two different people, Megan and Miguel, each wake up with a splitting headache. Megan thinks, "This is a

---

EXHIBIT 7.1

Negative Thinking

- "My pain is terrible!"
- "I can't bear it! How long must this go on?"
- "I shouldn't have so much pain. I don't deserve this."
- "I simply have to find some relief now!"
- "Why can't they make my pain go away?"
- "I'm going crazy! Where will this all end?"
- "I'm going to be an invalid. I can hardly do anything anymore."
- "I'm a burden to those around me."
- "I'll never get better."
- "This is going to get worse and worse. Maybe I'll go crazy."
- "No one else can ever really understand this pain."
- "I'll never be able to enjoy life again."
- "It's all my fault that I'm in this mess."
- "It's all _____ (for example, my boss's; fill in the blank) fault that I'm in this mess."

EXHIBIT 7.2

Realistic Thinking

- "The extreme pain is back again, but I know it is only temporary."
- "By relaxing my muscles, I can make my pain more bearable."
- "I can take a bit more rest today between activities. Tomorrow I'll get back on my regular activity routine again."
- "I want to do something pleasant or talk to somebody as a distraction."
- "I can keep my breathing as deep and even as possible and this will reduce my experience of pain."
- "Bad days are to be expected; we all have them. I might as well enjoy what there is to enjoy, even on the bad days."
- "I can stay in control of the rest of my life, even when my neck hurts."
- "Things are going slowly but in the right direction. I'm going to get better and better."

result of that busy day yesterday. I overdid it when I was exercising. I'll take a hot shower and take it easier today." In contrast, Miguel thinks, "This is the same pain my father described just before he had that stroke. I'm probably going to have a stroke. I must go to see the doctor immediately. But it is Saturday. What am I going to do?"

Megan now feels more relaxed, less distressed, and more in control. Miguel feels worried, discouraged, helpless, and dependent on others to feel better. As a result, for Miguel, the headache may worsen. By the time he gets to the doctor, Miguel will alarm the doctor to the point that she orders a CAT scan. Waiting for the test results, Miguel feels even more anxious, and his pain is almost unbearable. Fortunately, the CAT scan shows nothing abnormal. Both Megan and Miguel had a headache, but their reactions resulted in very different consequences.

We focus a lot on thinking throughout this book because the implications are serious. For example, faulty thinking often leads to poor sleep. How? When you focus on how bad things are, you are likely to feel even more miserable. Uncertainty, worries, and fear keep you from getting to sleep and staying asleep. Lack of sleep tires you out; you are fatigued, so you do less the next day. This inactivity further undermines your self-confidence, causes you to lose hope, and makes you feel helpless and depressed. Meanwhile, your pain is feeling worse.

If you have consistent difficulty falling asleep, and you are following a balanced activity and rest program described in Lesson 4, monitor your thoughts more carefully, particularly before you go to sleep or wake up in the morning.

To summarize our discussion so far, your negative or faulty thoughts about your situation can lead to emotions and more negative thinking that may not match reality. What you think quickly initiates what you feel both emotionally and physically. What you feel can then often lead to more faulty thinking and to what you do (or don't do) to help yourself. When you catch yourself in negative or faulty thinking, try to just gently label these thoughts as such and move on to a more realistic thought.

METHOD 2: BEHAVING DIFFERENTLY

The adage "If you can't feel a certain way, try *acting* that way for a while" means that it is easier to act yourself into feeling differently than feel yourself into acting differently. This does *not* mean being fake, as you will see further along in this section.

Consider the following: Have you ever noticed that when you feel you look good in the mirror, you tend to carry yourself differently, and people respond accordingly? On challenging pain days, one of our patients wears only his favorite ties when he volunteers at the library. These ties make him feel he looks good, even when he doesn't feel so good. When he's in the washroom, seeing the tie in the mirror reminds him to smile. Often, he will be complimented on his tie. But is it the tie or the smile?

Another patient of ours always serves herself lunch on her best china on days she feels the worst. It reminds her of the good things in life. Another patient forces herself to reach out at least once to someone else who is having trouble during her "bad weeks." Oddly enough, feelings often follow behavior, so you have more control over how you feel than you may realize. We are not suggesting it is simple, but even small things to make you feel better can make a difference in your thoughts, feelings, and behavior and how your body responds.

It may sound easier said than done, but your feelings don't have to determine your behavior. If you are feeling bad, you can still consciously decide how you will respond to your mood and pain. You can still decide whether you will think and behave positively or whether you will surrender to your feelings and think and behave more negatively. You have to pay attention to what you are thinking and move from unconscious automatic thinking to focused awareness and change. We're not saying it's easy. However, it is good always to be aware that although you can't control situations (including whether you have pain or what other people do and say), you do have some choices about how to respond inwardly and outwardly. And having choices is always a good thing because it means you can make good decisions as to how you respond. For example, when you feel sad, you can choose to pull the covers over your head. Or you can choose to unburden your heart or listen to music you love and allow your tears to flow or write about it in your journal. If you still feel sad, you can choose to feel bitter, or you can choose to act yourself into feeling different. You can make a conscious decision of how you want to respond to those sad feelings.

Afterward, you may find yourself thinking, "My sadness has had enough space to express itself; now I'm going to enjoy myself" or "My sadness is still here, but I will take a shower, do a few stretching exercises, and dress in my favorite clothes. I've listened to some sad music and gotten the tears out. Now I think I'll put on some more lively music." It may well be that as you do these things, you notice that you are singing or whistling along with the music and feeling better.

Even after funerals, or during the wake or visitation, people turn from their grief for a while to recall fond memories of and experiences with the deceased. Some groups even call their gathering a celebration of life, while also sharing their grief and loss. Often people are surprised to find themselves laughing at such times. But they shouldn't feel guilty about it. Life goes on. We can choose to live in the moment or dwell in the past or future.

To measure your success in this method, look at your behavior. For example, if you feel tired and listless, and you go swimming, you have had a successful day, whether or not your mood has changed. When you are in pain and call a friend to listen to her concerns, you have had a successful day, even if your mood has not changed. Success is not measured by moods or by pain but by the courage to take steps despite the pain. Remember the Serenity Prayer first mentioned in the introduction to Lesson 1—having the serenity to accept what cannot change, changing the things you can, and having the wisdom to know the difference between them. Always remember that you have choices.

Let's look once more at this idea of "acting yourself into feeling" for a person without chronic pain. People who lack self-confidence can be taught to look, walk, and speak like someone with confidence. If they practice those skills consistently, they feel more confident. A shy person who speaks softly and indistinctly and avoids the other's gaze is saying, without words, "I am not important. Don't pay any attention to me." He can be taught to speak up, look into the eyes of the person he is speaking with, and ask questions or give responses to show interest. As a result, he feels more outgoing. Try to remember that thinking differently and behavioral change lead to emotional change. In short, the feeling determines the behavior, and the behavior determines the feeling. Table 7.1 offers a few examples of how this can look in practice.

TABLE 7.1. Examples of Acting the Way You Want to Feel

Feeling	Spontaneous reaction	Result	Intentional action	Result
Sadness	Being still and alone	Depression	Talking, sharing	Processing, humor
Anger	Bottling it up	Aggression, rage	Telling what you think, telling what you feel	Peace, balance
Fatigue	Taking long breaks, being stuck in a rut	Exhaustion	Taking short breaks, doing energetic exercise	Improved condition
Pain	Feeling tightness, sadness, worry	Extreme pain	Engaging in relaxed behavior, positive outlook, feeling of control	Bearable pain
Shyness, fear	Avoiding contact, reacting with fight or flight	Phobia	Engaging in small talk, inviting others to socialize	Confidence

METHOD 3: UNBURDENING YOURSELF OF "MUST" AND "SHOULD"

When you tell yourself that certain things *must, should,* or *have to* be done, you cause emotional pressure and bodily tension and distress. If this tension exceeds a certain level, or if it lasts too long, it has a paralyzing effect. As a result, you may start to feel overwhelmed. Moreover, as noted earlier, these "musts" and "shoulds" cause more pain.

Unrealistic expectations of oneself can be a real burden. This is especially true for younger people with chronic pain who have families who used to rely on them for income, housekeeping, cooking, yard work, and so on. They feel that they "should" still be productive, even on challenging pain days. Releasing oneself from such unrealistic expectations can bring some relief.

For example, one of our patients felt he "should" continue a foreign language course he was taking for enrichment. That semester, the class was being held at another location. He drove around frantically because he could not find the new location. Finally, he saw a cozy little diner and decided (reluctantly) to ask for directions. Once there, the nice waitress and the happy conversations among the patrons inspired him to have a cup of coffee. He began to relax and realize that he was hungry. The aroma of the home-cooked meatloaf convinced him to order dinner. So what if he was late, he thought. Then, halfway through dinner, he decided to skip the class altogether. He felt slightly guilty but then thought, "The heck with that," and began laughing out loud to himself. It was a hobby, not a job! The whole evening was spent relaxing and enjoying the moment. The next semester, he decided to take a cooking course, which he enjoyed thoroughly.

Activities that you fear trying, feel forced to perform, or feel that you have to do are perceived as more difficult than activities you feel you have chosen voluntarily. For example, if you have certain nutritional goals for yourself, you can phrase your wish to eat more healthily as a choice, and you can reward positive behavior. Instead of saying, "Ugh, I have to eat more fiber," while selecting groceries, you can instead tell yourself, "Today I get to choose either broccoli or chickpeas. I haven't tried chickpeas—that's what I'll choose this time." Think about how you might reward your child for eating. You might say, "You are allowed to choose to eat from what's on your plate, and if you eat your meal, you will receive a nice dessert." The dessert offered might be something nutritious and also something the child likes (for example, sliced apples). This way, you can encourage your child to eat healthy, nutritious food. Make it clear that the child does not *have to* eat the food on his plate but is *allowed* to eat it. If, in addition to the french fries, he also eats the peas and chicken, he will then receive a dessert that he likes. The positive attention (reinforcement) follows the positive behavior. This may take time, but it is time that is not wasted on rewarding unhealthy behavior (such as nagging when your child refuses to eat— remember the laws of learning described in Lesson 6).

One of our patients, Bernie, who was too dependent on the opinion of others, found a stick-on decal that read, "What you think of me is not my problem." He stuck this on his smartphone case. It helped him begin to "act real" when he was talking with someone and not worry as much about their opinions of him.

Consider another of our patients, Lori Sue. She had been working with us for 6 months at the time of the events recorded in this story. Lori Sue had recently started working for an attorney after being out of work for several years because of a back injury. Her boss frequently waited until the last minute to give her an assignment. He then expected her to work miracles. On one Friday, once again, Lori Sue was given an assignment before lunch with an unrealistic deadline to meet. The work had to be completed by that evening. Lori Sue had social plans after work, which made things even worse.

She immediately began doing the research and making phone calls to collect and analyze all the information she needed to complete the assignment. She skipped lunch and did not take breaks so that she would get it all done on time. She felt her back strain from the buildup of pressure and from sitting in a rigid position. Lori Sue clenched her teeth, trying to ignore her pain and her feelings and found herself thinking,

- "My boss should have planned ahead better."
- "If I ignore the pain, I can get this done."
- "I can't afford to go slowly or take a break because my boss might think I can't do the job. I'll get fired."

By the end of the day, Lori Sue had not only an aching back but also a pounding tension headache and pain in her jaw from gritting her teeth all day. She canceled her plans and arrived home exhausted. She immediately collapsed into bed but had trouble sleeping.

On Saturday, Lori Sue remembered some of what we discussed together about coping with stress, and she began to think about her day in a different light. She came up with the following thoughts to replace the ones she had the day before:

- "My boss does not know what is reasonable and feasible for me."

- "Yes, it would have been nice if my boss had planned ahead better, but that didn't happen. My getting upset about that doesn't help me get through my work. I can't and will not manage this in this way."

- "Next time I'll stretch and relax in short intervals throughout the day, and the pain won't be so bad later."

- "Eventually, I'll have to let my boss know that I have a back injury. He won't think less of me. I'm good at what I do, and I always do my utmost to get the work done."

- "When we get to know each other better, I'll sit down and discuss how we might get the work done at a less hectic pace."

- "Because I missed my outing last night, I'll plan a nice weekend for myself. I'll call a friend after I have a leisurely breakfast."

What was your reaction when you read the first (Friday's) and then the alternative (Saturday's) set of self-statements? Did you feel a sense of pressure with the first statements and a sense of relief with the second? Also, did you recognize any of the self-care suggestions we have made in the previous lessons?

METHOD 4: STOPPING AT THE RIGHT TIME

If you push yourself too hard and feel you have to go on with an activity or commitment, you may do harm to the progress you have achieved. It is important to finish an activity while the pain is still bearable and to stop when it is at least not too painful!

This last suggestion implies that it is important that you have some control over pressure when other people are involved. This was an important thing that Lori Sue learned with her work assignments.

It applies as well to social situations. When you go somewhere with someone, for example, let them know that there is a chance you may want to leave earlier than they will. Ask in advance for the other's cooperation in this regard or suggest that you take separate cars. When you arrive at your destination (for example, the theatre, a concert, or a movie), try to arrange a seat that will enable you to leave easily if you find it necessary to do so. For example, at a theatre, reserve a seat at the end of the row near the exit. You will notice that feeling you are in control (therefore, able to leave) is liberating in itself and thus reduces tension.

When you are doing something "fun" that you are not enjoying, give yourself permission to stop (remember our patient who was taking the foreign language course). For example, staying at a party where you are not having fun because of your pain is not a useful strategy. For one thing, you may come to associate going to parties with having unbearable pain. Over time, you may find yourself avoiding social gatherings more and more. If, however, you leave when you are still feeling good, you give your body and mind the message that parties and socializing are fun.

Letting go of unreasonable demands and acting in your own self-interest allows you to feel more in control of your life and more independent of your pain. You can determine what is reasonable to do or not do, maintain a daily and weekly schedule, and take pleasure in all kinds of activities. You'll do these things not because you *should* but because you *want to*.

The risk of forcing yourself beyond your limits is greater in situations in which you cannot be yourself or you are not free to do as you wish. If you have a visitor, you might be afraid of appearing inhospitable if you ask the guest to leave. When you are back at work, you want to make a positive impression, and you cannot just walk away. This means that despite the pain, you do your utmost as long as possible until it becomes unbearable.

A result of this can be that visiting others or receiving a visit becomes an emotional burden. Working is associated with excessive pain, so you fear and avoid work. By now, you are probably starting to understand the power and pervasiveness of the laws of learning described in Lesson 6!

You need a safe climate. You can reduce your disability only if you have new, different, successful experiences with visits, work, and other stressful or emotionally charged situations. Only success in these situations will remove the pressure and tension and help you build self-confidence. Not working or not having others over for visits (in short, giving in to your pain) does not eliminate the pain or even reduce it. On the contrary, by giving in to the pain in this way, you reduce self-confidence and will likely experience even more pain (see Lesson 8 for more about pain and self-confidence). Do you have a lot of "should" and "musts" in your life? If you do, you might want to reconsider these and what effects they have on your thoughts, feelings, and behaviors.

METHOD 5: USING THE ABCD MODEL

The ABCD model can be a useful tool in helping you deal with pain and other stresses in your life. This is how it works:

- A is the *activating event* or stressor. It can be physical, emotional, social, or environmental. For our purposes, let's make *A* a muscle spasm in your back that keeps you from fulfilling a commitment.

- B is your *belief system*. This consists of your thoughts and attitudes about the stressor. For example, you might think, "Now I can't do what I said I would. My friends will think I'm weak and always unreliable. I can't do anything right anymore."

- C stands for the *consequences* of the activating event and your belief system. Consequences are often feelings or emotions. For example, as a result of the kind of thinking described previously, you feel down or depressed. You might also feel pain increase as you tense your back muscles.

- D is the way out. D means *disputing*, challenging, or questioning your negative belief system (the negative thinking that goes on after the stressor). This disputing, in turn, affects how you feel. For example, you might question whether your friends will really think that you are weak. You would certainly also challenge the statement, "I can't do anything anymore."

The ABCD model takes practice but yields extremely positive results over time. As you read this section, we suggest that you start using it whenever you catch an unhelpful thought. Don't worry about getting it right, but use this as an opportunity to pay attention to your thoughts and how they can play an important role in your pain and how it affects your life.

Whether you use a chart or simply jot down the As, Bs, Cs, and Ds, you will become acquainted with your belief system. Over time, you will more automatically and rapidly dispute the negative thinking that affects how you feel and gets in your way of living life. As you become more familiar with using the model, you will be able to use it without writing, simply working out the ABCDs in your mind.

Four Steps for Challenging Your Unhelpful Thoughts

Let's start with an exercise using the structured format. Try not to skip any steps (for example, don't jump from B to D).

A. First, write down a recent stressor or event that was followed by a pain flare-up. Keep this concise. A few lines are enough—for example, "I twisted in my chair while reaching for the phone and felt my back strain." If you're having trouble thinking of a stressor, go over the past 2 or 3 days when you felt pain. The more recent the stressor, the better able you will be to identify all thoughts and feelings.

B. Next, list all thoughts you may have had when your pain-related stressor occurred—for example, "My back is going out again," "I have to take up the slack and answer the phone for the other administrative assistant who's always out sick," "I thought my doctor said this wouldn't happen if I exercised regularly."

C. Third, jot down all the feelings you had right after the stressor. A key to identifying feelings (rather than thoughts) is that when describing feelings, you don't usually use the word *that*. If you find yourself saying "I felt that I . . .," you are likely describing a thought, not a feeling. For example, "I thought that the other secretary was faking" is not a feeling. However, it may contain hints to your feelings. It may contain clues to the feeling "I felt victimized." Notice that you don't say, "I felt *that* I was victimized." *That* typically doesn't occur in feeling statements. Other examples of how you might have felt in this situation are, "I felt angry and disappointed. Later I felt a bit hopeless." You do not need a long list of feelings. A few key ones will do. These feelings are the consequences of your thinking.

D. Finally, you will dispute the thoughts you listed in the second step. You will question whether "my back is going out again" is really the case. You might think instead, "My back hurts sometimes. Over time it will get better." Instead of, "My doctor said this wouldn't happen," you might think, "My doctor said that these events would happen less frequently if I keep to my pain management program." And finally, you might question whether the other secretary is *always* out sick. You might think instead, "She's out sick a lot. I wonder whether she's struggling with some physical or emotional problem."

As a result of disputing your belief, your feelings may change or become less intense. You may feel, for example, just mildly irritated at the other secretary. You may also feel less hopeless or sad.

As a result of having fewer negative feelings, you will likely be able to think of more positive things you can do for yourself. You might think, for example, "I'll do some relaxation exercises in the empty conference room for a little while"; "At lunch, I'll go for a short walk and have a chat with one of my coworkers"; "I'm going to trust that I will feel better over time"; "I'll seek some diversion, and I trust that I'll be all right again in a couple of days."

Table 7.2 shows a few more examples of situations in which the ABCD process can be helpful. We also include a blank downloadable form you can use for your own situations on the companion website (http://pubs.apa.org/books/supp/turk).

Try to work with the ABCD process. It may take some time until you feel comfortable with it. But don't let that discourage you. It should become easier with practice. Pay particular attention to the fact that the activating event does not lead to your feelings. It is your thoughts and beliefs that lead to these feelings. These thoughts represent your *interpretation* of an event. If you are having trouble disputing your beliefs, you might list several possible interpretations of an event and ask yourself, "Which interpretation of the event is most useful to me right now?" The example of Andrea described next illustrates the importance of the process.

TABLE 7.2. Examples of Using ABCD in Stressful Situations

Date and time	A Activating event	B Belief systems	C Consequences	D Disputation
9/14, 8:35 a.m.	Neck pain while driving	Oh, no, my neck is hurting again. I'll have to pull over and never get to where I'm going. I'll be asking others for rides now for weeks.	Fear, anxiety, feeling sick to my stomach	It will be okay. I may have to take a break and be late. I'll take it easy a bit later.
9/15, 10:30 a.m.	Boss angrily pointed out an error I made	How could I be so stupid? She probably wants to fire me. There goes my next promotion and raise. She is always expecting the impossible. I can't take much more of this!	Shame, anger, crying, heart racing	I feel bad that she yelled at me. She's probably having a really bad day. I'll talk to her some other day when we're both less stressed to see how we can make things go more smoothly in the office. Tonight, I'll listen to my meditation app and then text a friend to plan something.

How Andrea Used ABCD

One of our patients, Andrea, described a recent event that became a stressor. Let's see how she used the ABCD model to stay in control of her pain. This example also illustrates some of the stress-reduction and relational issues described in the previous lesson. See whether you can identify them as you read.

Andrea's partner, Jayden, was on a business trip for 4 days. Andrea had decided to go on an outing with a good friend the day before Jayden was due home, and she had a really good time.

That night she had to take out the trash. She carried a garbage sack that was too heavy to the curb and spent a restless night in pain (antecedent event [A] = lifting heavy bag). She thought, "I knew it—I threw out my back. I'm really in trouble now; it will probably get worse, and I'll not be able to get anything done for the next few days" (belief [B] = "It's my fault; it's going to get worse, and I won't be able to get things done").

When Jayden arrived home the next day, instead of greeting her warmly, Andrea began telling her partner all the negative things that had occurred while she was away. Andrea didn't even think to tell Jayden about the nice time she had with her friend. Jayden suddenly remembered that she had promised to fix their neighbor's broken porch light and told Andrea she would be right back. She was gone for over a half hour, and by this time, Andrea was fuming. (consequence [C] = Jayden ignored her, and she became angry).

Andrea decided to take a hot bath to calm down. She put some lavender bubble bath in the tub. As she relaxed, she isolated the event that led to her pain. Andrea realized that she was blaming Jayden for everything that went wrong while she was away. Then Andrea thought of her behavior when Jayden returned home. She had done the opposite of welcoming her partner. This insight led her to think about Jayden's decision to leave for the neighbor's house (disputing [D] = Andrea was blaming her back pain on Jayden for being away but then realized it was due to an isolated event and not Jayden's fault at all).

When Jayden came home, Andrea's pain was still there (although it had decreased after the bath). More important, however, her mood had changed, and so did her behavior. She asked Jayden about the trip. She went over to the sofa and began talking a little hesitantly. Andrea smiled as Jayden was talking, and she relaxed and took her hand. Jayden talked about how some of her colleagues were posturing during the event to make themselves look intelligent and important. They both laughed about this. By the time they had finished talking, Andrea noticed that her pain didn't seem as bad.

As you go through your day, like Andrea, note when you feel stressed or when you are feeling negative. You can ask yourself the following questions: "What events led up to my negative feelings?" "What did I believe or think about the event that may have led me to become upset?" "Are these beliefs or thoughts true and accurate?" "Are there other more constructive ways to think about what happened?"

SUMMARY

- Thoughts and feelings influence behavior more than knowledge and will-power. Feelings change and are often unreliable; facts don't change, and you can look at them in a helpful way.

- Do not ask yourself, "What makes me feel good?" Instead, ask yourself, "What things do I want to feel good doing?" Introduce the activities where you want to feel good in your life.

- Negative thoughts and feelings and being stressed have physical effects that can make pain worse. Remember, your thoughts and feelings can open and close the "pain gate." So, more positive thoughts and feelings may reduce the amount of pain you experience!

- Consider stressors or problems as challenges for which you can create a list of strategies, either on your own or with the help of your significant others. You can then try different strategies and see which one works best to resolve each type of challenge. Think of your success or lack of success with each strategy as a learning experience.

QUESTIONS TO CONSIDER

1. What do people expect from someone with chronic pain? What do others expect from you?
2. How do you respond to these expectations?
3. You are relaxed and friendly, despite the pain, or you start exercising again but still cannot go back to work. How do you explain this to your neighbor?
4. Do you expect and demand a lot of yourself? How can you change this?
5. What actions can you do to influence your pain levels?
6. What thoughts and beliefs open or close the "pain gate" for you?

HOME ACTIVITIES

1. Over the next 3 days, try to jot down in your journal or notebook all the thoughts that occur to you concerning your pain. Note when and where these thoughts occur.

    Try to act as an objective observer while writing down your thoughts. In other words, try not to censor or debate your thoughts; simply write down all the thoughts that come to you. Remember that it takes practice to become familiar with your particular brand of thinking. Automatic think-ing is lightning fast. The first day you will likely miss some thoughts. But on the second and third day, you should have quite a list.

    Go over your thoughts and try to label them using the list of common thinking errors. Don't be concerned if some don't fall into a specific category. Just underline them and go back to them sometime later. This practice will be invaluable as you get to know your patterns of thinking.

2. Take the thoughts that you recorded in the previous activity and choose one category of thoughts that recur (for example, catastrophizing). You may want to choose the type of thoughts that occur most frequently. Any time one of these kinds of thoughts comes up in the next week, use your journal or notebook to write down statements to dispute these thoughts. After you become adept at disputing one category of thoughts, work on the second category of thoughts.

   The following are a set of thoughts our patients have found useful in disputing their automatic thoughts. See whether you can use some of them. Then add some of your own that will be useful in the future.

   - "I can cope."
   - "It's no one's fault that I am in pain."
   - "Relax, I can manage my pain."
   - "I have managed this situation before, and I can manage it again."
   - "Most people act out of their own motivations. It's unlikely they really meant to hurt my feelings."
   - "I am learning new coping skills each day."
   - "The pain comes and goes. I can outlast it."
   - "No one thinks less of me because I have this pain."

3. If you like a more structured approach, you may want to construct a table in your notebook or journal and keep a diary of stressful situations using the ABCD model. Try to catch your thoughts in stressful situations, even if these are not directly related to your pain. We have included some examples in Exhibit 7.2 to give you an idea of how to do it.

Gaining Self-Confidence

Life is not easy for any of us. But what of that? We must have perseverance and above all confidence in ourselves. We must believe that we are gifted for something, and that this thing, at whatever cost, must be attained.

—MARIE CURIE

If you have worked through all (or most) of the lessons in this book so far, you may be feeling better, if not physically, then at least emotionally. Hopefully, if you are working on your SMART goals, you are also seeing some positive effects in other areas. (Remember, a SMART goal is specific, measurable, achievable, relevant [personally meaningful], and timely.) Your life is different and, although you may not even be aware of it yet, the seeds of self-confidence have been planted.

Every day you follow the program working on your goals, practicing the different exercises and coping skills, it's like caring for your garden. Eventually, your self-confidence will become apparent to you, like the first flowers arriving in spring.

With time you are becoming more and more resilient—that is, you have been increasing your ability to overcome the effects of pain and the impact of chronic pain in your life while maintaining your normal emotional, physical, and social functioning. Resilience is not a final state but a dynamic process that can develop and grow over time with your effort. As you become more resilient, pain will become less prominent in the foreground of your life. It will be more like background noise that is bothersome but does not stop you from living a satisfying life. You will have grown from being a person coping with pain to a person thriving *despite the pain*. This is all because you have

- listened to your body and your thoughts and taken the right steps to respond to these signals,

145

- developed and achieved reasonable (SMART) goals,
- paced your activity and rest cycles,
- increased the variety of pleasurable experiences in your life,
- improved your relationship with others,
- learned to think yourself into feeling and acting better, and
- persevered through the program, practicing what you have learned and persisting even in the face of any difficulties that may have arisen.

Not only are you developing confidence in yourself and becoming more resilient, but you are also developing confidence in others and the future in general. In this lesson, you will learn how to enhance some of these skills to build your confidence further. We'll start with a brief recap by way of questions to consider and then build from there.

HAVE COMPASSION FOR YOURSELF AND YOUR BODY

- What are you able to do today? It is important to distinguish daily what your body prevents you from doing (what you are physically incapable of doing) and what your thoughts and feelings limit you from doing. This helps you to make friends with your body rather than attacking it with thoughts such as, "My back is always acting up and hindering me" (therefore, my back is the enemy). It is important to listen to your body, even if what you hear is not positive. But remember that listening to your body and giving in to discomfort are two different things.

- Are you beating yourself up today with self-defeating thoughts? In the past, you were tough on yourself, berating yourself in your thoughts when you were unable to do all you expected of yourself. If you are feeling down today, you may be whipping yourself. Ask yourself why. You may be giving more than you have to give and thus feel depleted. Or you may be having thoughts such as, "I'm such a burden to others. I have to ask for help today, and I'm ashamed that I can't do it myself." These thoughts are self-defeating, and they make you feel even worse. You know yourself better now, so you can most likely quickly identify these types of unhelpful thoughts (see Lesson 7 to review some of the common self-defeating thoughts and ways to dispute them).

- If you are having a challenging day today, how can you keep your head above water? At some level, even on the most difficult days, you know that you can only work *with* your body, not *against* it. Think of your body as a child. Care for it as if you were taking care of a child. You nurture the child, but you do not coddle her. You listen to your child, not only when the child is happy and healthy but also when the child has pain and is sick, don't you? Do not be afraid of listening to your pain. It doesn't mean the pain will take you over. You are still in charge. You have the knowledge and skills to take on the challenges that confront you.

Learning to Accept, Respect, and Love Yourself

You can only grow to accept, respect, and yes, love yourself as you are. Loving yourself is not holding yourself up to some ideal standard of what you would like to be at any given time, although you might have a reasonable and realistic standard toward which you want to work. Try to remember that everyone who does their best at any given time has a right to self-acceptance and respect. Judge yourself on commitment and effort, not on results. When you do your best, even though it is not perfect or "ideal," you still have to give yourself credit. You may view yourself as a patient when you are having a challenging day, but what if you viewed yourself first as a person, a person worthy of your respect and goodwill despite having limitations because of your pain? A person with diabetes does not think of him- or herself as a patient, assuming most days they go about their day with food preparation and/or glucose monitoring steps simply built into the normal routine. In the same way, all people with chronic diseases, including chronic pain, have to view themselves as a person first.

Self-acceptance is the important first step in learning to love yourself. The second step is to invest your time and energy in your well-being before any other priorities. This investment does not mean you are being selfish. It means you are being responsible. Only when you feel good about yourself do you have anything available to give to others. Only when you respect your needs can you then respect the needs of others.

We discussed acceptance early in this book. Here, it is important to elaborate on that topic because you will have difficulty building confidence in and loving yourself unless you fully understand what acceptance entails.

The Process of Acceptance

First, acceptance is an ongoing process. It is not a final state that can be achieved for good. Acceptance provides a moment-to-moment atmosphere that permits the possibility of change for the better. From the time your chronic pain began, the journey of acceptance has been a process of moving through several stages, sometimes in a circular fashion rather than straight through. These stages include:

1. Denial of limitations. In this early stage, you act as though nothing has happened. You act as if there is no real problem. You hide your condition from yourself and others, presenting yourself as feeling better than you really do. You may use painkillers, alcohol, or other substances to continue denying your pain problem.

2. Rebellion against and anger about limitations and pain. In this stage, you are aware of the pain and the existence of a problem, but you fight this awareness. You may push your body as if it is a machine. You may frantically call on all kinds of specialists and feel misjudged and misunderstood by everyone. You keep fighting even if it causes you more pain.

3. Despondency, depression, and passivity. In this stage, you may view the pain problem as unsolvable. You feel helpless and hopeless and do not see a way out. You may avoid responsibilities or experience sleeplessness during the night and excessive fatigue during the day. You may increasingly turn to alcohol and other drugs. You may just want to crawl into bed and feel helpless and hopeless.

4. Openness to adapting to new circumstances and to learning new things. In this stage, you become more open-minded. You decide that you have a problem (or problems) but that there may be solutions. You may buy a book such as this one to gain some understanding and guidance. You may begin to feel more hope, more control over your life. You begin to feel better about yourself, and as a result, you interact with people differently. Instead of seeing setbacks as failures, you see them realistically, as part of the process of living with chronic pain.

5. Acceptance. As a result of going through Stages 1 to 4, you gradually come to accept your body, your situation, your chronic pain, and yourself. Instead of fighting, you make peace with your body and yourself. This acceptance is a process, so in some days, hours, or moments, you may be more accepting than others. It is important to realize that you move back and forth between these stages. That is why we emphasize that acceptance is an ongoing process. You will find yourself at different stages of this process at different points, even when you are following the advice in this book and taking good care of yourself. What stage do you feel you are in today, at this moment? What is important is how you respond to whatever stage in which you find yourself.

It is also important to emphasize what acceptance is *not*. Acceptance does not mean that you no longer feel pain or that you no longer see the consequences of having chronic pain. You are still aware of limitations. Not every day is an easy day. Not everyone responds in the way you would like. You don't always accomplish everything you planned. Acceptance is not pushing yourself beyond realistic limits, and it does not involve setting unrealistic standards ("musts," "oughts," "shoulds"). It is also not doing less than one is able. Acceptance is not just giving in or giving up, either. Acceptance means just that—that you accept the positive and the negative without needing to deny or exaggerate either. Remember one of the concepts in the Serenity Prayer from Lesson 1: Develop the serenity to accept the things that you cannot change. Acceptance, however, does not mean giving up. Recall the rest of the Serenity Prayer—it asks for the courage to change the things you can and, importantly, the wisdom to know the difference between what you can change and what you cannot.

BECOMING YOUR OWN BEST FRIEND

Before you can truly accept appropriate support from others, it is crucial to become your own supporter, your own best friend.

Perfectionism is the enemy in becoming your own best friend. You may not think of yourself as a perfectionist, but you may be surprised. Do you criticize yourself silently when you make a mistake? Do you silently say things to yourself such as "That was dumb" or "I should have known better"? Are your sentences littered with words like "should" or "must"? When others do things to help you, do you sometimes feel resentful because they don't do them as you would if you could (remember the case of Janet and her children we described in Lesson 5)? These are all telltale signs of perfectionism.

Perfectionism is the enemy because it is not fair to demand more from yourself than you can achieve. Nobody is born a perfectionist. Usually, you learn to become a perfectionist early in life. Sometimes you learn to expect perfection in some areas but not in all areas.

In the past, you may have heard, "Make sure you make a good impression" or "What would the neighbors [relatives, neighbors, teachers, boss] think?" Or you may have belonged to a highly productive organization where you encountered much more skill in being self-critical than in being self-confident. One of our patients learned to push herself so hard that when she won a red ribbon (second place) in an art competition, she felt bad because it wasn't a blue ribbon: "I *should* have come in first." Note the self-degrading "should" in her thinking.

Unconsciously, such experiences become internalized. That is to say, they become part of yourself, who you think you are, and how you think about yourself and others. Without even being aware of it, you may be operating under the beliefs "What others think is more important than what I think of myself" or "Only the best is good enough."

Take Pride in Your Uniqueness

Think a moment about your uniqueness. What is unique about you and how you think, feel, and act? If this is difficult, think about some funny quirk, something positive. Or think about the size and shape of your eyes or your laugh or lifelines (don't even think of them as wrinkles). It is unlikely anyone else has the same shade and shape of eyes or the exact laugh or placement of lifelines. Try to improve the way you talk with yourself, given your uniqueness. Even limitations can be considered unique. When you try and don't succeed, how about saying to yourself in a friendly way, "That was a fair try. Trying is more important than succeeding. I like and respect myself for trying. I'll probably do better some other time, with more experience, more practice, more information." Try not to compare yourself with others or with your "former self." You should like yourself for who you are and who you may become!

If a person is continually watched, observed, and evaluated by others, he or she experiences a lot of stress and distress all the time. If you are constantly doing this to yourself, you will cause yourself unnecessary problems or magnify small ones. You'll behave more naturally and feel more relaxed when you are not worried about how you measure up to some arbitrary and unachievable standard or when you are not measuring yourself against others.

If you grew up with brothers, sisters, or cousins, do you remember how it felt to be compared in a negative light? It was unlikely that it made you feel good about your uniqueness or motivated you in a healthy way. For example, if you felt driven because of how others compared you with your peers, it was not a healthy form of motivation.

Instead of comparing yourself with others or with your idealized self, find a way to be proud of yourself for your efforts as well as your accomplishments and for who you are. Seeking and finding your way will give you confidence. See how it feels to proudly say, "I did it my way, and it worked out better than I expected" or "I did better by my own efforts."

Don't Try to Earn Love

Love is a gift freely given and freely received. If you think you must do your best to be loved, your thinking is confused (remember what we covered in Lesson 7). When you try to earn love, you do yourself and often others a great injustice. In fact, you are setting yourself up to fail! Your lovability is not determined by what you have or what you *achieve*, but who you are. Babies and puppies don't have much and don't achieve much but are loved nevertheless.

Self-love is most important. Self-love is more about who you are at a point in time, what positive qualities you would like to achieve, and the efforts you make to achieve them. You can grow and alter who you are. Think for a moment: What kind of person do you want to be? What qualities go into being that person? How can you work toward achieving those qualities? It is only fair to charge yourself for your efforts and not your results. Can you love yourself in the process?

Although the next question may seem a bit unpleasant, it can be useful to ponder. How do you want your family and friends to remember you if you die before them? Try not to think of proving something to them (or if you do, you may want to consider this question: What do you want to prove and to whom?). It's satisfying to be able to say to yourself, "I don't have to be as good or better than others to be perfect. I just have to be myself, the best I can be." Life, for everyone, is an evolving process.

You may think, "I may not be as good as I would like to be, but I can work to improve; however, I can accept myself as I am now, with my imperfections and my limitations and also with all my unique characteristics. That is how I want to be thought of and how I would like to be remembered."

Control the Things You Can Control

As we discussed earlier in the book, many things in life are not under our control. But it is helpful to take charge of things that you can control. The following statements may be helpful in that regard. Try saying one of them to yourself each day, and see how they fit.

- My situation is not responsible for my mood. I can redirect my thoughts and change my mood.
- I am not my appearance, height, intelligence, income, health, or accomplishments. I am me, and that is enough, but I can grow.
- What others think of me is not what is most important. What is more important is how I think and feel about myself.
- I am not responsible for other people's moods or their happiness, but I can be a positive influence on both.

There is no doubt that when you have chronic pain, you need assistance at times and support always. But often, you may feel diminished and dependent when this occurs. Most people are unaware of it, but this is not a problem of dependency, it is a problem of pride. All of us are dependent on others—*all* of us. From the barista at the coffee shop to the most powerful politicians and wealthiest persons, all of us rely on others. An African proverb says, "It takes a village to raise a child." And it still takes a village to live a good life when you're an adult.

If you have difficulty accepting the interdependence of people, think about electricity. Aren't we all dependent on electricity and roads and schools and on the people who provide these services? Aren't we dependent on farmers and fishers and ranchers for our food, construction workers and plumbers for our houses? "Yes," you may be thinking, "but that's a condition that is shared by everyone. I have to ask for help some days just to get the mail."

First, let's look at what makes it unpleasant to you when tasks and responsibilities that used to be yours have to be taken over by others. Does it make you feel as if you are not indispensable or that you can easily be replaced? Do you begin to feel "less than" or worthless?

Society plays a big role in glorifying (false) independence. If you have bought into this, you are likely to feel sad or angry or depressed when you need help. You may start taking these feelings out on others, who seem so independent to you. You might begin telling them that they are not doing tasks properly or the way you would do it. If your friends and family tell you not to worry, that they will take care of something, do you behave even worse? If they seem frustrated at being interrupted, do you feel ashamed or angry?

These are all signs of false pride. It is nothing to be ashamed of, but it is something to work on. For many people, receiving is more difficult than giving.

Does this ring a bell for you? Could you consider that when people help you, you are giving them a gift as well? Feeling helpful is a good feeling. Can you work on receiving help graciously and showing appreciation?

If this is too difficult, find a way to help others first. See how you feel when you make a phone call and listen to someone who feels lonely or sad or anxious without needing to get anything in return. See how it feels when you offer a piece of information to someone who can use it, perhaps through a note in the mail or a quick text message.

Then, the next time someone helps you, try to remember the good feeling you had helping someone else. Even if your helper is grumpy, don't assume that helping you is not helping him or her. Be gracious anyway. If your friends and family tend to help too much, you can ask them to involve you as much as possible. If you can't help in doing the task, you may be able to help in the organization and planning. Also, emphasize to them that it is helpful to you if they would sometimes ask for your advice, counsel, and support. They may have as difficult a time asking for help as you do! Choosing to be interdependent means trusting in others.

Ask for Help

In a dance with one partner leading and the other following, the partners have to trust each other. With your family and friends, it's important to think through what you want and need before you ask them to do something for you. Often, people think they want something concrete when they really want some time and attention. Sometimes people think they want attention when they want someone to fix a meal or do the laundry. So, take the time to ask yourself what you want. Then, find the courage (yes, it takes courage to ask for what you want) to tell them directly. Gently tell the people in your life how they can help and how they can play an important role in your life.

If you still have difficulty with asking for help, you may need to rephrase the way you are asking. Here are some ways our patients have asked for help:

- "Would you be so kind as to . . .,"
- "Would you possibly be able to help me . . .,"
- "May I please ask you to do something . . .,"
- "I would really like . . .,"
- "You would do me a great pleasure by . . .," and
- "I would be grateful to you for. . . ."

Try to remember when one person is unable to help, to think of someone else. It is important to have a range of people whom you can call on for assistance. Interdependence does not mean you relate to just one person. It means having a network of people to whom you can give and from whom you can receive.

You can be rightfully proud of yourself when you have learned to ask for help graciously, when you have learned to express appreciation for help, and when you have been able to accept "no" for an answer just as graciously. These capabilities will add to your self-confidence and improve relationships with friends and family.

Stand Up for Yourself

Many people find it hard to stand up for themselves. Lack of self-confidence, feeling unlovable, fear of conflicts, and a lifetime of habitually not asserting oneself are all obstacles to this important capability.

People who don't stand up for themselves tend to avoid conflicts. They may say "yes" when they mean "no." They may not agree with something, but for the sake of peace, they give in. However, in the long run, they are not able to hide their true feelings. Then, when hurt feelings and frustrations eventually become too much to contain, they are likely to be expressed in the form of an outburst of anger.

The people around them are frightened, and they may be frightened too. They may feel bewildered and embarrassed. They may think, "This is not like me. I don't like that person who just came out. I must never do that again."

When people with chronic pain are not assertive, the people around them start to treat them differently, more as a patient than as a person. People no longer say what they think but what they think the patient wants to hear (recall the discussion in Lesson 5). Everyone tries to mind-read, which never works. So, family and friends may avoid the person with chronic pain. Everyone eventually begins to wear a mask that is not natural and is exhausting for everyone.

If this description seems to fit your situation, you may begin to feel that you are not an equal partner in the relationship. Others may feel you are no longer their support and refuge. To begin to change this, it is important to learn how to express yourself and make your position clear in each situation that requires this.

When something bothers you or when people are pressuring you to do or say or feel something you don't want to, it takes courage not to cave in. But, if you want to have a *real* relationship with the people around you, and if you want to feel better about yourself, you must begin to say no. You must begin to challenge people when they behave in ways that are not helpful. Let's focus on saying no (see Lesson 5, Table 5.1, comparing assertive, nonassertive, and aggressive responses).

In the beginning, this will be hard. You may be awkward. People who are not used to asserting themselves often say no more harshly than they intend when they first try out the word. Think of ways you can say no in a respectful but clear way by reviewing situations in the past when you said yes when you meant no. How might you have responded differently?

In the beginning, you should start with the easiest situations in which to say no in your own way. Gradually work up to more difficult situations. As you do this, you will gain confidence in yourself and feel more in control of the things that are under your control (namely, your decisions about where to go and what to do).

Balance, Balance, Balance

In all the situations described previously, it is important to seek balance. For example, in asking for help, try not to move from one extreme (for example, doing it all by yourself) to the other (for example, asking others do everything). You can ask people to do certain tasks for you temporarily until you can improve your functioning. You can begin to do small things for yourself that you used to ask others to do for you. But, remember, some days, no matter how well you have followed this pain management program, you may need more help than other days.

Don't start saying no to everything when you never said no to anything before. Don't try to be assertive with everyone at first. Take your time. Skills and capabilities need time to develop.

LEARNING TO SOLVE PROBLEMS

Many people assume that self-esteem is a feeling. Actually, it is a result of acting in certain ways: nurturing yourself, communicating well with others, being assertive, following through on commitments (especially to yourself), and effectively solving problems, to name a few.

Here we focus on problem solving. Problem solving is not a natural ability. It is learned. The first step in learning is to begin thinking of problems and conflicts differently. If you always see things from the other's point of view, try thinking of the problem or conflict from a different point of view (for example, an objective observer of the situation). If you always see things from your point of view, try mentally walking in the shoes of the other person involved in the conflict or problem. Most problems with other people are communication problems. It's amazing to learn how often we misinterpret other people, and they misinterpret us.

One of our patients found it helpful to write about such problems in letters (unsent) between herself and the other person. First, she wrote about what happened (the specific behaviors, not the interpretation of the behaviors) and how she felt (not thought) about it. Then, she did the same from the point of view of the other person. This helped her stay open-minded and kept her from "dumping" her feelings on the other person. Next, she visualized the benefits of having addressed the problem or conflict constructively.

Exhibit 8.1 provides a list of stages and questions that are helpful to consider in solving any problem, particularly when you write your answers in your notebook or journal.

Solving the Problem of Pain-Associated Distress

Let's look at this structured problem-solving method with regard to pain-associated distress. First, redefine the problem as something that is *affected* by the pain, not the pain itself (usually a feeling, thought, or behavior). For

EXHIBIT 8.1

The Steps of Problem Solving

Step	Question or action
1. Problem identification	What is the real problem or concern?
2. Goal selection	How do I feel? What do I want?
3. Generating alternatives	What can I do? What else can I do?
4. Decision making	Which alternative seems best?
5. Implementation	How can I do this? Do it!
6. Evaluation	Did it work (solve the problem)? If not, what went wrong? Return to Steps 1 to 5 as often as needed.

example, you might redefine the problem as a conflict with your partner over scheduling or distress about a lack of social activities in your life. Define this problem in specific terms.

For example, in the case of a conflict with a partner, the problem is not "getting along with my partner" but "adjusting our schedules to meet my partner's needs and any limitations that I have."

Next, define what you feel and what you want in specific terms, as well. For example, in the case of a lack of social activities, you might write, "I feel lonely and not part of life. I want to have more people and activities in my life."

Then, generate some ways of dealing with the problem. Brainstorm a list of at least three ways you might help solve your problem and don't edit your solutions before you consider them. Some of our patients have found it helpful to imagine how others in similar circumstances might respond if asked to deal with a similar problem.

From your list, for each proposed solution, evaluate the advantages and disadvantages from your point of view (and, in the case of a conflict with a person, from the point of view of that person, as well). Rank the solutions in the order in which you think they might be most likely to solve the problem. Don't think of right or wrong but what you think would be likely to be the most successful to the least successful.

Consider how you might go about putting this solution into practice. Again, it might be good to brainstorm a list. Think through how you might engage in activities to lead to a good outcome, one that resolves the problem.

Then, try out what you believe would be the best and most realistic approach to solving the problem.

Finally, evaluate what happened. Was it successful? Partially successful? Did it fail? If it wasn't fully successful, what might you have done differently? Do you think that one of the other alternatives you generated might have worked better? Why?

Don't expect that everything will go the way you hoped or that the problem will be completely resolved or resolved in all the situations where it tends to crop up. If the problem continues to bother you, return to Steps 1 to 5.

For example, you may have to redefine the problem. You might add new approaches to your original list of problem-solving alternatives.

In any case, remember to give yourself credit for making an effort to solve the problem constructively. For example, you might say to yourself, "I've made a good start. I'm not going to sit back and hope or wish the problem would go away. I'll reward myself for trying, for making an effort, and then go back to think through the problem again."

You can learn a lot from people who have already attained success (not perfection) in their lives. The approach these individuals take has been studied, and it has been found that successful people possess certain characteristics and observe certain practices. These are described in the sections that follow.

Autonomy

Autonomy requires learning to set your own (SMART) goals. You can involve others, but the final responsibility for your goals and your choices is yours. It also involves letting go of meeting others' expectations of you and being less sensitive to what others think of you. This may be harder than it at first appears, but it is an attribute worth working toward.

Appropriate Risk-Taking

This involves being prepared to take risks. People with this characteristic focus more on what they have to gain rather than what they have to lose. Reynolds Price, the author of many books of fiction but also an account of his serious illness, *A Whole New Life*, learned to take this approach when he became ill. Like other successful people who exemplify this characteristic, Price did not take unreasonable risks, but he did learn to know and accept himself, to be realistic, to weigh outcomes, to appreciate his need for support, and to make choices based on these factors.

Realism

Successful people are realistic without being drawn into pessimistic or overly optimistic thinking. They don't aim too high or too low. They pick themselves up when they fail, and they evaluate what they might do better next time. They don't expect to run the marathon unless they have trained systematically.

Present Orientation

Successful people do not dwell in the past, which they consider "history." They are continually active in making realistic plans for the future and who they want to become eventually. They take the initiative in making these plans become a reality by experimenting in the present. They can benefit from their previous efforts (history), in that they can learn from their efforts and the results to inform future efforts.

Focus on Possibilities

Successful people focus on possibilities. Instead of rehearsing the problem over and over, they are most involved in thinking about solutions. They develop talents that enable them to meet challenges, and this makes life seem like a challenge that is interesting and exciting.

Strive for Success

Successful people have the courage to strive for success, even when they encounter major obstacles, such as pain or serious illness. They realize that hope alone is not enough. Instead of focusing on fear of failure, they focus on the hope of success and the discipline and life skills needed for it. They hope for the best and prepare for the worst. Mistakes are seen as learning opportunities, rather than reasons to despair.

Resilience

Successful people who are living with chronic pain have to become resilient. To do this, they have to make use of their resources, learn from their experiences and from others, and adapt to challenges. They do not rigidly stick to self-defeating strategies. They grow from them.

This lesson has reviewed some of the material covered in earlier lessons and outlined a number of other ways to regain your self-confidence. Reread the lesson when you are feeling down or a bit hopeless. Each time you read it, you may take in a little more.

SUMMARY

- You can only learn to live with pain if you regain confidence—confidence in yourself, others, and the future. The necessary steps for regaining confidence are:
  - taking yourself seriously;
  - listening to what your body has to tell you;
  - understanding that you can work with your body, but you cannot fight against it—that is a battle you will lose; and
  - accepting the facts.
- Acceptance makes change possible. It is a process of four stages:
  - denial, acting as though nothing is changed;
  - aggression, fighting against better judgment;
  - depression, feeling helpless and hopeless; and
  - acceptance of yourself as you are now, taking adequate measures.

You may cycle through the stages of acceptance multiple times as your health status or other circumstances change, but hopefully, with experience, the harder stages will go by more quickly or become easier to bear.

- We are all dependent on others in some way—even the president and billionaires. Being able to do less does not mean being less. You can still contribute meaningfully to other people's lives through your attention, interest, and involvement.

- You are worthwhile and worth the necessary investments you make in yourself, such as rest and space. Speak kindly to yourself.

- You can make your needs, wishes, and desires known to others—if you do this, you will not have to wait until others figure out what you need and what is best for you.

- Practice the six steps of problem solving and apply them to your pain-associated distress. Congratulate yourself for making an effort, even if your problem isn't resolved at the end of the process.

- Allow yourself to be led by the hope of success and not by the fear of failure. Be alert to ways you can experiment and take responsible risks, setting your targets incrementally higher. Learn from the past, but focus your energies on the present and the abilities you have today.

QUESTIONS TO CONSIDER

1. From what sources do you draw your sense of self-respect and confidence? How is your self-confidence undermined? Which people have you given a lot of influence over your peace of mind?

2. Looking back at the stages of acceptance, where would you say you are now regarding your chronic pain? Where have you been so far, and what did it feel like when you realized you were in a new stage?

3. What attributes of successful people do you share?

HOME ACTIVITIES

1. List two problems you have been struggling with recently. Use the steps in problem solving described in the lesson to work on these. Write out the steps and your responses in your journal or notebook.

   Put your solution into practice, pay attention to what went well and what did not, evaluate what went right and what went wrong, and consider alternatives if the desired outcome was not achieved. Make sure you reward yourself for trying, even if the outcome is less than you hoped it would be.

2. Think of a conflict or a problem you have recently had that involved someone else. Use the same problem-solving steps that you did in the previous activity and record your work in your journal or notebook.

3. If you are unassertive, reread the section on assertiveness here and in Lesson 5. Try saying no to a person with whom you feel safe. Then, as your confidence in this capability grows, begin saying no to people who tend to intimidate you.

Putting It All Together

Be not afraid of life. Believe that life is worth living and your belief will create that fact.

—WILLIAM JAMES

Pain is an important messenger, and pain management is the critical skill you need to decode your pain's message and be resilient despite the pain. That, in a nutshell, is what this lesson—indeed, the entire book—is all about.

As most dieters know, the initial pounds are easier to lose than the later ones. However, keeping weight off for good is more difficult than losing it in the first place. Being able to develop a plan, stick with it, and modify it as needed, dealing with setbacks as they occur is the most important thing you can do after your initial attempts to get started have finally resulted in measurable progress.

Before you started this book, you may have assumed that your pain was solely the result of some physical damage in your body. We have tried to emphasize that physical factors definitely are involved. However, as you have seen while progressing through the lessons, other elements contribute both to your pain and the effect of pain on your physical and emotional functioning.

In this lesson, we weave together all the new insights, skills, and strategies we have shared throughout the book. We have added a few more, as well, such as the effect of the past on the present, problems with motivation, and the finer points of setting goals. Because knowledge is power, we want you to have as much power as you can with regard to your pain and your life. We want to help you feel resilient.

PAIN: PAST, PRESENT, AND FUTURE

Previous pain experiences can influence your current experience of pain and the thoughts and feelings associated with that pain. If you ever had to leave a job under adverse conditions (for example, you were fired, the company was transferred), you probably will never forget the emotions you experienced. Even after several years in a new workplace, if problems arise, you are likely to experience, consciously or unconsciously, a level of anxious arousal. It is as if stressful memories predispose us to experience anxiety in situations we encounter later but that seem similar. If you have had surgery, some emotions (and possibly physical effects) are likely still there. These serve as reminders of the distress you experienced. In other words, when you experience pain in the present, you are likely also to experience the effects of memories from previous pain experiences.

However, memory and pain cause distortions. If your pain is severe now, you may recall your previous pain as being less severe. If the pain you feel now is mild, you may recall that the pain you used to experience was worse. Your present pain becomes the anchor by which you judge what your pain used to be like and what you anticipate it will be like in the future. These memories feel as if they are true, regardless of objective reality.

Your present pain can also influence what you anticipate ("What if this pain gets even worse?") and consequently cause you to limit your activities to prevent pain in the future. However, as we have seen since Lesson 1, anxiety and worry open the pain gate, so these moments of anticipation are important to recognize as such.

It may also be the case that your feelings of pain are telling you something about the present—the here and now. Your body does not protest without reason. Maybe there is too little security, support, and balance in your life, or it feels that way. It could be that the relationship between your coping resources and your burden (what you have to bear) is out of balance. Numerous other factors in the present can cause your pain to increase—family problems, emotional upset, worry, lack of understanding from your significant others, financial or work problems, or inappropriate activities, to name only a few we have previously described. The pain in the present is telling you to take stock and shore up your resources.

Even experiences from the past that are unrelated to pain can influence your reaction to pain. The laws of learning we discussed in Lesson 6 do not just apply to physical pain. The laws of learning help shape our character and, therefore, our habitual ways of being and behaving. Are we flexible or rigid? Are we comfortable with some emotions (for example, sadness) but not others (for example, anger)? Did we learn from and do we resemble our parents, family members, or other strong authority figures in our ways of dealing with emotions? We learn not only from our own experiences but also from what we observe, and this information will have an impact on what we expect and believe and how we behave.

We are aware of and can remember only a small proportion of these previous learning experiences. It is especially the negative or distressing experiences that we push out of our conscious memory as a matter of survival. Most of us cannot be consciously aware of all the sadness, loneliness, fear, and pain we have experienced in our lives. Nevertheless, a negative atmosphere growing up, illnesses in our families, traumatic experiences, and poor coping models (for example, how did family members deal with diseases and pain?) do leave their mark—the more intense the experience, the more pain in the family, the greater the influence.

Fear of being dependent on others or feelings that you are not allowed to be weak or sick can be a result of experiences you had growing up. For example, if, as a child, you had to carry a lot of responsibility to survive, you may find it difficult later as an adult to let go of control with confidence. How might this same pattern be at work in your present life?

Let's say you did have to carry too much responsibility as a child. Now, you may have difficulty asking for help. After you have hurt yourself doing something you weren't ready to do, you might also find yourself saying, "Why am I so stupid?" "Why did I have to do it all on my own?" or "I should have asked for help." If you were consciously aware in the present of all that had happened to you in the past, you would know that your pattern of independence is understandable. There was likely a time when you had to do it all by yourself. You had to do this to survive and function. In other words, in the past, there were circumstances in which that independent streak was appropriate, but now it may be causing you difficulty.

Did anyone in your family have a chronic disease or chronic pain? How did they deal with it? What did you learn? Do you think how they responded has any effect on how you are dealing with your chronic pain? You may not be aware of it, but your prior experiences—even those you can't recall—do have a powerful influence on how you think, feel, and behave now.

YOU HAVE THE POWER TO CHANGE

The good news is that, as a more consciously aware adult, you have the power to create a safe and positive environment in which you can learn more adaptive skills. Some people assume that "you can't teach an old dog new tricks." But studies have shown that people not only can change but also do change throughout life. Development over time is inevitable. People can and do change even in their 90s and beyond!

Think about how your pain may have influenced your personality. Many people we have treated have told us, "I am not the same person I was before the start of my pain." Positive changes can happen as a result of pain as well as negative.

You may know people who claim they can't change. It is true that people differ in their degrees of ability to change. Each person has different learning histories that shape who they are. The "hardware" (the brain) is roughly the same for most people. But the "software" (past experiences, thinking, feeling, and behavior patterns) is uniquely different for each one of us. Anyone suggesting that they cannot change is making an excuse. Making this excuse takes away their responsibility for doing anything to improve their lives and leads to dependency—a place where they are stuck, have given up, are helpless, and can't be blamed. They are seeking and deserving of attention and sympathy for their plight.

Initially, you were "programmed" by your genes, family, and community environment. As you grew up, you began to develop your preferences, goals, and styles of thinking, feeling, and behaving. The initial software programs, although never entirely erased, can be modified with life experiences and one's behavior.

Many people dislike particular programs or patterns they see in themselves or others. Alcoholics, chain smokers, drug addicts, and pain *patients* (in contrast to people who have pain) may intensely dislike many aspects of themselves or their current lives, but they feel helpless to change. They have yet to take responsibility for their lives.

As the author James Allen stated,

> Each of us is the architect of our personality. Not the circumstances, not the problems, not the pain, but how we deal with it determines our sense of happiness. Happiness is not the absence of pain and cares.

Taking Charge of Your Response Patterns

Before you experienced chronic pain, you were used to functioning in a particular way. After the pain, you became used to functioning differently. Both lifestyles were a set of habits, a part of who you were or are. Most people are attached to their habits, even if they are not good habits. What you are familiar with feels good, and there is always a certain resistance to change. As we said, habits are sometimes formed during particular periods of your life, and they may simplify life because we don't have to pay attention to them. These habits may be difficult to let go of when you reach another period.

Pain is similar; it can result in habitual thoughts and behaviors, and that is why we have stressed changing your thoughts, feelings, and behaviors, even if doing this takes you out of your comfort zone. If you do not adapt constructively, you can make life harder, even unbearable, for yourself and those around you, as in the case of Janet, Glenn, and their children that we described in Lesson 5.

Even good habits can become destructive when followed too rigidly. For example, we have stressed that it is a good idea to spread your work, chores, physical activities, and errands over the week rather than trying to accomplish them all in one day. Organizing your activities in this way offers important advantages. You accomplish just as much, if not more, but with less strain.

However, if this good habit becomes the driver and you the passenger, even a paced schedule can become a problem. For example, if you have found it helpful to tidy the kitchen thoroughly on a Saturday (rather than trying to clean the whole house that day), and you have a challenging day on Saturday, you may feel that you have to tidy the kitchen anyway. You may have decided this not because it is necessary, but because it is Saturday. You push yourself. Your habit, rather than your real need, has become the driver in your life. Flexibility must be a part of a well-balanced life.

If you want to change *bad* habits, a few strategies can be helpful. Ask yourself what this habit helps you maintain (fear, pride, perfectionism?). If these feelings are difficult to work through, you might find it helpful to see a counselor for a few sessions. However, what is not helpful with a difficult habit is simply to excuse it by saying, "That's just the way I am." That excuse will give you a temporary out, but in the long run, it will defeat you.

What is most helpful is to prioritize the habits or sets of responses you want to change and choose one to change at a time using the methods we have outlined in this book.

Motivation

In earlier lessons, we described why and how to get motivated to make changes. Let's call that *Motivation 101*. This is the next level in learning about that topic. Let's review first.

The amount of effort you are willing to put in to reach any goal is your motivation. The strength of your motivation is determined by the following:

- whether your goals are SMART (specific, measurable, achievable, relevant [personally meaningful], timely);
- the clarity of your goal: Exactly what do you want?
- the attractiveness of your goal: What are the benefits to you?
- the perceived and actual feasibility of your goal: Is it possible or realistic, given your current limitations?
- your skill level: Do you have the knowledge and skills necessary to achieve your goal? and
- your willingness to persevere: Do you have the courage to continue despite occasional setbacks?

Many people with chronic pain say, "I would do anything to get rid of the pain." If you have the will to change, good intentions are not sufficient—you have to be willing also to make an effort and persist even if progress is slower and more difficult to achieve than you would like and even if you experience setbacks. If you are having difficulty putting the lessons in this book into practice, you might review the preceding list to see whether motivation is a problem for you. What is holding you back?

The Seasons Change, and so Do You

Try to keep in mind that what you find enjoyable today, this week, or this month may not always be enjoyable or as enjoyable. The things that bring us joy are not constants. Sometimes, social contacts bring us joy; other times, solitary pursuits (for example, hobbies, prayer, meditation) bring us greater joy. Some people use enjoyable activities to motivate themselves to do things that aren't enjoyable (such as phoning a friend after they have taken a walk that they didn't look forward to). But after a while, they find that the prospect of the phone call no longer helps them over the hurdle of walking when they don't feel like walking. Then, it is time to think of new ways of bringing oneself joy.

Other ways of staying motivated include becoming more knowledgeable. We have emphasized throughout this book the importance of both others' knowledge about pain and your personal knowledge of pain. It helps to update your knowledge bank from reputable sources when you are feeling bored with your pain management program. We have listed some resources you might find of interest in Appendix C.

But it is also helpful to gain knowledge in any area to keep your mind sharp and your interests lively. It is best to do this when you are not in a down period or having a challenging day. It's hard to push yourself to learn a new skill or body of knowledge when things are not going as well as you would like.

Instead, when things are going well, or you are having a good day, begin to think about what you would like to learn to do or what you would like to study. Some television can be relaxing, but a daily overdose of television can be deadly to mind and spirit. Perhaps you have always been interested in the history of quilting or sports but have never found the time to explore this. Perhaps your interests are in archaeology or poetry. Don't feel you have to have training or a college education to explore your interests. Just begin where you are and build knowledge and skills that will later serve as resources when other areas of your life are not so good.

What does this have to do with pain? When pain is unavoidable, distraction can be one's most useful ally. However, you must become acquainted with your ally when you are not in pain to feel comfortable turning to your ally when distraction is truly needed.

THE MECHANICS OF GOAL SETTING

Motivational problems sometimes stem from not knowing how to set goals. Although we cover the basics of this topic in Lesson 2, there are some finer points you may want to consider.

As we noted in Lesson 2, setting goals is important. You should set goals that are specific, measurable, achievable, relevant (personally meaningful), and timely.

Most people need both short-term (today, this week) and longer term goals (several months, even years) to feel successful. It is helpful to formulate your goals in terms of daily, weekly, monthly, several-month, and annual goals.

It is also important that you formulate your goals in terms of effort, not in terms of results. This is because we have control over our efforts, but we do not have complete control over the results.

Place your goals, especially your daily, weekly, and monthly goals, in a prominent place, so you are reminded daily of what you are trying to do. Periodically review your monthly and annual goals to remind yourself of what you are working toward and your progress to date. Use this information to help motivate yourself. If you are not making the progress you planned, consider why and make changes in the goals or your behaviors that might be needed.

Making copies of the activity, relaxation, and progress charts provided early in this book are useful tools to keep track of progress toward goals. These, too, can be posted in prominent places while you are using them. As you fill in each chart, consider filing the old ones in a three-ring binder containing tabs for each month to help you keep track of your changes over time and your thinking and behavior. Most office supply stores offer a binder with a clear front cover pocket where you can insert a picture, photo, or paper with inspirational words on it to remind you of your goal.

As you see progress in moving closer to achieving your goals, your motivation will increase. When you see connections between helpful patterns and positive benefits, your motivation will increase as well. The sense of accomplishment will help build self-esteem. And viewing progress, even if not always as much as you would like, can serve to reinforce you for your efforts and motivate you to stick with your plan to self-manage your pain, related problems, and your life.

Our patients have taught us that goals work like magnets. The closer they get to them, the stronger the attraction.

SUMMARY

- Pain can tell you something about the past, present, and future. When you uncover the factors that make your pain worse, you will be able to manage it more effectively.

- Be what you want to be. Try to change things you do not like about yourself. Practice the desired behavior by doing it as often as possible; allow the new behavior to become your second nature.

- If you are never satisfied with what you have done, do not say, "That's just the way I am." You can change your habits. Choose a balanced approach by starting with something small and recording when and how you started to notice the change. Plan how you will maintain the change and alter your living environment, to the extent you can, to support your new habit.

- The strength of your motivation is determined by the clarity, attractiveness, and feasibility of your goal and by your attributes. If you want your treatment program to become a practical reality, ask yourself, "How clear are my goals, how attractive and how feasible is what I want, and which attributes do I need to implement this program?"

- Your goals work like magnets—the closer you get to them, the stronger the attraction. Visualize clearly how you can include the correct balance of optimal effort, beneficial rest, and stimulating recreation in your day, week, and year plan. Formulate your goals as specifically as possible. Place them in a prominent place like on the door of the refrigerator, on the mirror in your bathroom, or next to your bed.

- If you become discouraged with the speed of your progress, you can review your tracking charts to see how you have moved forward.

- Pain is a message. You need a well-defined approach to managing it. Listen to your body and replace the overwork or the anxious inactivity with activities that quietly build up your physical and mental reserves. When you can tackle life again and enjoy it, you will know and feel, "I am in control of the pain and my life!"

QUESTIONS TO CONSIDER

1. What factors from the past influence your pain?
2. What factors in the present influence your pain? What can you do about this?
3. What factors in the future influence your pain? What can you do about this?
4. What is the one habit or pattern of responses that you would most like to change? How will you do it?
5. Which of your self-motivation tricks no longer work for you? How can you update them so that you are making more progress toward your goals?

HOME ACTIVITIES

1. Where is the most pain in the present? Plan an approach to control and reduce (not necessarily to eliminate) the pain in the present.

2. Think about a habit of yours that has been difficult to change. Then, list some of the ways to motivate yourself that we describe in this lesson. Pick one or two and try them for at least 6 weeks (it takes at least 6 weeks to change an ingrained habit). At the end of that time, record in your notebook or journal how and why you were successful in changing.

3. Consider approaching your stubborn habit as a problem and applying the problem-solving steps discussed in Lesson 8.

4. If you have not tried any of the activities so far, consider why this is so:
   - Are you going through a demanding time, but you will do the activities as soon as you can catch your breath?
   - Do you tend to put yourself last on your list of priorities and perhaps need to rethink that?

- Do you tend to procrastinate and need to work on that?

- If you have discovered particular problems with regard to your past that may be contributing to your difficulty in practicing this program, write about these in your journal or notebook.

- If you continue to have difficulties with problems you identified despite your efforts, you might want to consider short-term counseling with a therapist who is familiar with pain management as well as with general problems of the past influencing the present.

Maintenance and Coping With Setbacks

I don't believe in failure. I believe every setback is an opportunity to learn, regroup, get stronger, and try again.

—ROSELYN SANCHEZ

Success in managing your pain depends on your capacity to adjust, make changes as needed, and continue despite obstacles encountered along the way. For chronic pain, we have seen that changes may be necessary in just about every area of life—your daily activity and rest habits, the way you choose to think about your pain, your mood, and the way you relate to others, to name only a few.

Even when you have made changes, you will likely see that some changes are hard to stick with or that some changes, although easier to stick with, lose their effectiveness over time. This may be because your health status changes or because a new resource for coping becomes available to you or because of some other change in your circumstances. The important thing to remember here is that change is a process, not a single discrete event.

In this lesson, we emphasize *maintenance*, which is the critical last step in this pain management program. We review the three most important pain management principles. We also discuss how periodic lapses, relapses, and setbacks are normal and to be expected—in fact, they may be inevitable. They should not be taken as failures, but opportunities to explore and problem solve (see Lesson 8).

THE TOP THREE PAIN MANAGEMENT PRINCIPLES

Pain control comes about when you are reasonably able to exert yourself physically despite some discomfort or pain. Likewise, pain reduction occurs when you can relax despite the pain and divert your attention to focus on other things.

Principle 1: Bringing More Physical Activity or Exercise Into Your Life

Exercising within your limits can be beneficial both physically and mentally. The keys to success in this regard are being active *regularly* and *consistently*. Having a plan that matches your abilities, limitations, and interests helps with this. Our patients have taught us that if they establish a schedule and stick with it, they invariably begin to feel after some time that pain and pain-related problems occur less often and less intensely.

Principle 2: Ensuring Sufficient Relaxation

Acceptance and peace can't coexist with struggle and tension. Our patients have taught us that balancing activity and rest and finding time each day for relaxation and enjoyment are crucial to pain management.

Principle 3: Bringing More Diversion and Fun Into Life

Pain needs competition diversions that help you focus on the things that are going well in your life or that create opportunities for well-being mentally and emotionally. One pain expert, Bill Fordyce, observed, "Pain does not hurt as much to those who have something better to do." This changes the scene from pain in the foreground and life in the background to life in the driver's seat and pain in the back seat. Our patients have taught us that boredom and being stuck in a rut are roadblocks to successful pain management and regaining control of their lives. Most people find the first two principles simpler (note we do not say "easy") to implement. The third principle gives many people the most problems.

Consider the case of Fernando. Fernando had significant pain problems, and when his wife suddenly died, he was barely able to provide essential care for his three children. One evening, his son approached him about helping with a school project. Fernando sent him away—he was exhausted from the day. However, his son kept on badgering him. Troubled by guilt about not paying attention to his children, Fernando decided to try to get involved with his son. He helped his son break the large project into manageable segments. Fernando worked on the project with his son for half an hour before they went to bed. Fernando found that while spending time with his son, he did not focus on his pain. Fernando also felt a sense of satisfaction—he was able to keep his wisecracking son on task, while also enjoying his son's humor and stories about classmates. For the next several nights while spending time with his son—helping him find good Internet resources, finding the stash of art supplies, and doodling with colored markers while his son worked on a draft—Fernando was pleasantly distracted. The pain did not disappear completely, but it faded into the background. It was no longer the focus of his attention.

In Lesson 3, we described relaxation exercises, and we noted that you cannot pay attention to everything at the same level at the same time. While you are reading this page, you may not be aware of your air conditioner or heater fan making sounds in the background, your watch on your wrist, or your socks on your feet. Now that we mention these, you may be more aware of them, but as you pay attention to them, you are not able to pay as much attention to what you are reading.

You need the healthy balance that is realized by social contact, creativity, and, yes, fun. Fun, as Fernando learned, can be as unpredictable as the weather. One has to decide to "go outside" of oneself to discover it. Developing hobbies, stimulating creativity, deepening social contacts, playing games, becoming adventuresome, talking, laughing, and even reading and writing can bring fun and color into your life.

For each person, what is enjoyable will differ. Some find satisfaction in quiet pursuits, whereas others like the hustle and bustle of being in a crowd. If you are having difficulty with this pain management principle, remember to seek activities that fit you, but don't be afraid to step out of your comfort zone once in a while and try something new. Here are some additional ideas to get you thinking about diversions that might work for you:

- Are you especially interested in material things? Are you practical? Activities such as crafts, car or motor repair, model building, sewing, woodworking, and quilting are practical and creative as well.

- Do you enjoy learning new things? Activities such as chess, bridge, crossword puzzles, and Scrabble often appeal to people who like to stretch their minds and learn new things. Other food for the mind can be found in libraries and on the Internet. (Be cautious with the Internet, however—there is a lot of "junk food" online as well.) Mentally, you can go on voyages of discovery to far away, foreign regions; you can go back in time, to earlier civilizations; you can share the thoughts of the great thinkers; or you can bury yourself in countless subjects or specialize. Especially when you are less able to be continuously physically active, enriching your mind can be a powerful antidote to pain.

- Do you have artistic interests? Activities such as drawing, painting, music, drama, and literature are examples of artistic interests. You don't actually have to create to be creative. You can simply enjoy the creations of others. Being artistic includes being as well as doing. If you haven't considered such activities before, try to have an open mind. Try out different areas. There is a saying that is apt here: "The unknown is unloved."

- Are you interested in social activities? Volunteer work of all kinds, club memberships, community center activities, special interest groups, or classes are examples of fun that might appeal to you once you've given them a chance. If you have a talent for organizing or volunteering for service clubs, political parties, community action groups, and the like, there are many opportunities for you to have fun doing what you do best. The main thing is to ensure that you have people in your life and that you keep meeting *new* people periodically. If getting around town is too difficult, write letters, telephone people, ask them to drop by. People are unlikely to visit unless invited. Take the initiative on your good days; later, even on your bad days, you will find social companionship comforting.

- Do you like to work with numbers? Activities include starting collections, volunteering to be the treasurer for an interest group, joining or helping set up an investment club, and so forth.

- Do you have an interest in nature? Are you interested in everything that lives and grows? You might choose to put some effort into container gardening, keeping an aquarium or terrarium, keeping a pet bird or cat (but not both!), putting together a herbarium, fishing, and participating in ecological activities, among others.

In Lesson 4, we included some additional examples of different activities that were suggested by our patients. By no means should these be viewed as a complete list of interests and activities. You may have some ideas that are enjoyable that we have not even hinted at. Many others we list will be of no interest to you whatsoever. What is important is for you to have a list of enjoyable activities that fit you and from which you can choose on a regular basis.

To sum up, when you can no longer perform what used to be your "normal activities," you will likely have a sense of empty space in your life. If nothing pleasurable is found to replace these activities, negative emotions such as irritability, depression, or sadness may fill up this space. Sometimes it takes a serious jolt to be released from these emotions. Then, unexpected sources of strength and energy are found. The case of Eileen shows how this happened to one of our patients. We hope you won't wait for such an event to begin enjoying life and unearthing strengths and talents that you may not even know you possess!

Eileen's Resilience

Eileen took part in our pain management program and was determined to improve her life. However, she felt stuck. No matter what she tried, she felt her situation deteriorating. Walks became shorter; she started using a walker and eventually needed a wheelchair.

A few months after starting our program, her son was involved in a serious car accident. During Eileen's difficulties, her son had always been a great support. Now he needed her help. To her surprise and the surprise of those who knew her, the new task, the new demands, released unexpected energy. Eileen was able to help her son, first by making phone calls for him. Then, she found she was able to prepare meals once or twice a week. Finally, she began doing most of the shopping herself too. She used her mobility devices but was able to get around with much less pain. Even as her health condition changed, and she used the wheelchair more of the time, Eileen was able to uncover abilities to adapt that she never knew existed. Once her son recovered, Eileen began to volunteer at a children's hospital, reading to children and counseling parents about how to cope.

The What, How, and When of Staying Involved in Life

When you have a clear picture of the kinds of activities that interest you, it is important to make a choice and a plan. Ask yourself specific questions:

- What do I want to do?
- How will I accomplish this?
- When will I start?
- What do I need to do to get going?
- What problems might get in my way?
- What can I do about potential problems that I anticipate or that arise unexpectedly?

It often helps to tell others what you want and plan to do daily. Seek advice and encouragement from others. Each evening, take a look at what pleasurable activities you included in your day. And ask yourself, How far did I get with my plans? Do my plans need adjusting? How might I bring even more pleasure into my daily life?

MANAGING FLARE-UPS

Most of our patients experience periodic episodes of worsening pain, occasional sleeplessness, morning stiffness, and distressing thoughts and feelings. These flare-ups are usually temporary and, if managed well, are followed by continued improvement. When flare-ups occur, it is important to take an active approach to managing them. At first, you may feel distressed that the pain has returned or gotten worse, and you may be discouraged with your progress despite your efforts. You might worry that the pain has returned full force, will never remit, and might get worse. In your darkest moments, you may feel that all is lost—that the skills you learned in this book have been of no use whatsoever. During flare-ups, you might recall what we said about Murphy's Law: "If something can go wrong, it will." And let's not forget Mrs. Murphy's commentary on Murphy's Law: "Murphy was an optimist!"

But seriously, let's look at the causes of flare-ups. Flare-ups are sometimes caused by identifiable aggravating factors. A weekend doing too much yard work or the physical stress of repetitive motion (for example, too many hours at the computer) may be followed by increased pain and stiffness. Emotional stress, such as conflicts with family or friends, may also aggravate the level of pain and lead to sleeplessness. Certain weather conditions may set off a flare-up. However, many times, flare-ups occur with no identifiable cause. In these cases, it is best not to spend too much time analyzing what caused the flare-up because this may actually increase the pain. If you do identify specific factors that clearly aggravate your pain, you can possibly reduce them in the future by avoiding or limiting certain activities, planning to deal differently with conflict, and so on.

Before the next flare-up occurs, the most important thing you can do is to develop a personal *flare-up management plan*. In Exhibit 10.1, we describe a typical plan.

Note that this is only one example. You are unique, and you need to develop plans specifically for you. It can be helpful to go over your plans with a nurse, doctor, or physical therapist. This kind of planning is called *relapse prevention* in many fields, including pain management.

Planning Ahead

We've also included a blank form you can customize with your flare-up management plan (see Figure 10.1). On the book website, you will find a downloadable form (http://pubs.apa.org/books/supp/turk).

After a flare-up, it is important to rest and recover (for a reasonable, limited time while still maintaining activity using your pacing skills). It is also important to review what was effective and to commend and comfort yourself for having weathered the increased pain.

What to Do During a Flare-Up

But what do I do during a flare-up? This is a reasonable question. During a flare-up, relying on your newly developed qualities and skills learned

---

EXHIBIT 10.1

Sample Flare-Up Management Plan

- Change activity—add enough rest cycles to decrease activities by one half.
- Cut back on physical exercises by a certain amount—check with a physical therapist to determine the amount.
- Over several days, gradually increase activities up to level before the flare-up.
- Practice relaxation and controlled breathing exercises twice as often as before the flare-up.
- Increase the use of other pain-coping skills such as distraction, imagery, and positive thoughts.
- Increase the frequency of relaxing activities.
- Inform family that you are having a flare-up and what you will be doing about it.
- Tell significant others what they can do to help you during the flare-up.

FIGURE 10.1. My Flare-Up Management Plan

If I have a flare-up of my _____, I will do the following:

Change	How I'll implement the change
Increase number of rest cycles per day	From _____ to _____ rest cycles Other:
Ask PT how to change or cut back on exercises	PT advice:
Gradually increase activities	Increase _____ to _____ times/minutes per day Starting on this date:_____ Next increase_____
Relaxation and breathing Imagery and positive thoughts	From _____ to _____ relaxation/ controlled breathing cycles Positive thoughts and images to incorporate:
Who I need to tell about the flare-up, how they can help	I will tell _____ They can help me by:

PT = physical therapist.

throughout this program is critical. Remember that pain and distress are an inevitable part of life. Remembering that you are not alone in the world of chronic pain is helpful, as well. And most important, remember that you are resilient and can reclaim your life even with some reasonable accommodations and the occurrence of setbacks.

Acceptance of pain when you are having extremely high levels of discomfort is never easy. But our patients have taught us that if they try to observe the pain without trying to change it, they feel better than when they are frantically seeking control over the pain. They have told us that it is better to observe their thoughts and feelings than to act on them impulsively. They have told us that acceptance may not decrease pain, but it may decrease their suffering.

Keep in mind the saying "Pain is necessary, but suffering is optional." Pain and suffering are not the same. Pain is the physical hurt you feel; suffering occurs when you tell yourself lies about pain (such as that it will never go away) and judge yourself harshly for having or causing your pain. Suffering occurs when you blame other people who are not to blame or when you try to control people, places, or things that are not under your control. Pain is unavoidable at times. Suffering is a result of the lack of acceptance of that pain and associated feelings and emotions. Suffering also occurs when you forget that there is more to life than even intense pain. Suffering decreases by engaging in pleasurable activities that soothe and satisfy your senses, such as listening to music, stroking a pet, watching a relaxing show on television, burning a candle with an aroma you enjoy, having a cup of your favorite fruit or ice cream, or getting or giving a massage (even a foot massage can be highly pleasurable).

When you find out that you can put your flare-up management plan into action, and you can bring rest, harmony, and enjoyment back into your life, despite pain, then you know that you are accepting life on life's terms. Although you may be in pain, you will not necessarily be suffering!

A FINAL WORD

Your investment of time and energy in this pain management program and your commitment to your well-being have made you a different person than you were when you first started this book. Regardless of flare-ups, setbacks, and other unexpected challenges, you have become resilient, you have reclaimed your life, and what you have accomplished is irreversible!

It is our fervent belief that the information and guidance we have provided in this program, and most important, your diligence and efforts, have increased your resilience—your ability to adapt successfully in the face of the challenges posed by your pain, the related stress, and the difficulties you have and to bounce back when you encounter challenges.

Despite your efforts, you will continue to experience some pain. Any chronic disease, including chronic pain, will extend over time. Hopefully, you will experience reduced amounts due to your efforts. We encourage you to return to review the different lessons in this book periodically any time you feel a refresher will be useful.

We have shared a tremendous amount of information with you. We hope to hear from you about what worked and what didn't! Remember, we're in this together! We will learn from you and your experience, as well.

The following are the key points of this pain self-management program. You might want to copy it and place it someplace where you will see it frequently so that it can serve as a reminder.

KEY POINTS TO REMEMBER

- Be alert to the erroneous myths about pain:
  - Pain is *not* a reliable signal of injury. Hurt and harm are not equal.
  - The absence of injury or disease does not mean that your pain is not *real*—*all pain is real*. Your pain should be taken seriously.
  - There is no pill for every ill. Also, "when in doubt, cut it out" is not a useful way to treat chronic pain. Lack of activity feeds a downward spiral.

- Even if you have had pain for a long time, there is much you *can* do about it—you are neither helpless nor hopeless.

- You are a *person*, not a *patient*!

- Know your limits—balance overload and underload to find the optimal activity load for you.

- Move it or lose it! But exercise smarter, not harder.

- Maintain a regular exercise plan that gradually increases until you reach an optimal level, then stay with it. Keep charts where you record your exercise.

- The pacing of activity and energy is important, so balance activity and rest (relaxation).

- Maintain a regular sleep schedule.

- Practice relaxation and controlled breathing exercises daily.

- Give yourself permission to engage in pleasant activities, and plan for them as part of your everyday routine.

- Communicate with significant others—rely on *sharing*, not *mind-reading*.

- Be aware of the laws of learning and the role of attention, anticipation, and fear.

- Thoughts, feelings, behavior, and body are related. The *pain gate* can be opened or closed by each of them.

- Change painful thoughts into realistic ones. Don't worry about what you should, must, or ought to do—instead think about what you want to do and the steps you can take to achieve those goals.

- Accept yourself and your limitations; the new you may be different from the old but not worse.

- Reward yourself for your efforts and not just the results.

- Expect relapses, setbacks, and challenging days, but do not let them defeat you!

- Be yourself, act like yourself, and like yourself so that you can take good care of yourself! And finally, be proud of yourself for making an effort to take control of your pain and your life. We believe that your efforts are worthwhile.

We return to the Serenity Prayer with which we began this book and that we hope you have heeded:

the SERENITY to accept the things you cannot change,
the COURAGE to change the things you can, and
the WISDOM to know the difference and thereby;
to reclaim your life despite your pain!

HOME ACTIVITIES

1. Make three plans:

   - A plan to systematically become more active over time (indicate what, when, where, how much, and for how long).

   - A plan to bring even more fun and relaxation into your life (indicate what, when, where, how much, and for how long).

   - A plan to deal with inevitable flare-ups (that is, your relapse prevention plan). List the options, skills, and techniques you can use. Be as specific as you can. Place this in a prominent location so you can refer to it immediately when you need to.

2. Schedule a check-up with yourself on your pain and follow through with your appointment.

After you complete the final pain self-assessment, go back to the ratings you noted after Lessons 1 and 5. Remember to think about your behavior, thoughts, and feelings during each of the weeks that you recorded your pain and responses. Reflect on any changes you have made so far. Are your changes making a difference in your pain?

PAIN SELF-ASSESSMENT

Now that you have completed *The Pain Survival Guide*, it is time for a checkup to see how things have changed. As you provide your ratings to the following set of questions, compare them with when you started (your ratings at the end of Lesson 1) and midway through the program (your ratings at the end of Lesson 5).

Circle your rating on the scales that follow and compare them with the ratings you made after Lesson 1 and Lesson 5.

1. Rate the level of your pain **AT THE PRESENT MOMENT**.

$$0 \quad 1 \quad 2 \quad 3 \quad 4 \quad 5 \quad 6$$

No pain   Very intense pain

After Lesson 1   After Lesson 5   Now

_____   _____   _____

(As needed, review Lessons 1 and 3 for refreshers.)

2. On average, how severe has your pain been during the **PAST WEEK**?

$$0 \quad 1 \quad 2 \quad 3 \quad 4 \quad 5 \quad 6$$

Not severe   Extremely severe

After Lesson 1   After Lesson 5   Now

_____   _____   _____

(As needed, review Lessons 1 and 3 for refreshers.)

3. In general, during the **PAST WEEK**, how much did your pain interfere with daily activities?

$$0 \quad 1 \quad 2 \quad 3 \quad 4 \quad 5 \quad 6$$

No interference   Extreme interference

After Lesson 1   After Lesson 5   Now

_____   _____   _____

(As needed, review Lessons 2 to 4 for refreshers.)

4. During the **PAST WEEK**, how much has your pain changed the amount of satisfaction or enjoyment you get from taking part in social and recreational activities?

$$0 \quad 1 \quad 2 \quad 3 \quad 4 \quad 5 \quad 6$$

No change   Extreme change

After Lesson 1   After Lesson 5   Now

_____   _____   _____

(As needed, review Lessons 3 and 5 for refreshers.)

Some of these questions can also be found on the West Haven-Yale Multidimensional Pain Inventory (Kerns, Turk, & Rudy, 1985).

5. During the **PAST WEEK**, how well do you feel that you have been able to deal with your problems?

0   1   2   3   4   5   6

Not at all   Extremely well

(As needed, review Lesson 8 for a refresher.)

6. During the **PAST WEEK**, how successful were you in coping with stressful situations in your life?

0   1   2   3   4   5   6

Not successful   Extremely successful

After Lesson 1   After Lesson 5   Now

_____   _____   _____

(As needed, review Lessons 3 and 5 for refreshers.)

7. During the **PAST WEEK**, how irritable have you been?

0   1   2   3   4   5   6

Not irritable   Extremely irritable

After Lesson 1   After Lesson 5   Now

_____   _____   _____

(As needed, review Lesson 7 for a refresher.)

8. During the **PAST WEEK**, how tense or anxious have you been?

0   1   2   3   4   5   6

Not anxious or tense   Extremely anxious or tense

After Lesson 1   After Lesson 5   Now

_____   _____   _____

(As needed, review Lesson 7 for a refresher.)

Have these numbers gone down, remained the same, fluctuated, or gone up? If they have gone down, great, but if they have fluctuated or gone up, don't be discouraged. This is not unexpected as people improve at different rates. It would be worth your effort to try to identify what factors may have affected your ratings. You might want to review the material in the Lessons that are most relevant, as noted after each question (we provided some reminders of the most appropriate lessons related to each question) and check out some of the sources listed in the appendices in this book.

Common Treatments for Chronic Pain

In this appendix, we present a list of common treatments and therapeutic approaches for chronic pain. It is not intended to be a complete list of all alternatives but includes those most frequently used or discussed, listed in alphabetical order. Many of the approaches can be used in combination. As you explore this list and the evidence we have included, there are several things to keep in mind.

1. Many studies published in the professional and scientific literature report positive outcomes for various treatments. These studies may be carefully carried out, but they are single studies. When possible, you should seek additional research on the same treatment to see whether the positive results are confirmed. Cochrane regularly publishes systematic reviews of the evidence for the benefits and safety of different treatments for specific pain conditions (see the Cochrane Database of Systematic Reviews: https://www.cochranelibrary.com/cdsr/about-cdsr).

2. We note that the long-term benefits of the treatments listed are largely unknown. That does not mean that they are not effective in the long term, only that research studies have not been conducted to evaluate these longer term benefits (or harms that might occur over time even if initially beneficial). The majority of the studies follow patients provided with the treatments for only relatively brief periods—3, 6, or 12 months. Rarely are any studies published that follow patients beyond 1 year after completing a treatment that is prescribed. So the effects of these treatments beyond 1 year are unknown.

3. Many of the treatments listed, as well as new treatments to help patients with chronic pain, are continuing to be developed and evaluated. Thus, the information we provide here and the evidence mentioned are only current as of the date we are reporting them (August 2019). New information will be forthcoming, and you should stay alert.

4. Be cautious of media advertising and testimonials from a single individual or few individuals who have received some benefits, paid public figures (for example, actors or prominent sports personalities) who appear to endorse treatments and who have no special knowledge of scientific research, or paid health professionals who may be predisposed to be positive in their endorsements.

ACUPUNCTURE

Acupuncture is a method of pain and disease control discovered in China almost 5,000 years ago. In acupuncture theory, imaginary lines on the body (called *medians*) represent internal organs and other parts of the body. Points on these lines are thought to connect different parts of the body. One or more of these points are stimulated by the insertion of an acupuncture needle. When the needles are placed in the skin, the practitioner may gently twirl the needle by hand or by an electrical current attached to the needles. Some needles are stimulated for brief periods of 10 to 20 minutes and then removed; others are left in for longer periods. The needles used are thin and solid, and virtually no pain is felt when administered by a qualified practitioner. The U.S. National Institutes of Health is currently studying the effectiveness of this treatment for various conditions. At this time, the results are somewhat mixed, with some studies showing short-term benefits but others reporting no significant benefits (Lam, Galvin, & Curry, 2013). As with any treatment, if you decide to have acupuncture, be sure to seek a qualified practitioner.

ANALGESIC MEDICATION

There are three primary classes of pain-relieving ("painkilling") medications (referred to as *analgesics*):

- Nonsteroidal anti-inflammatory drugs (NSAIDs). Many pain-alleviating treatments in this class can be purchased without a prescription (e.g., aspirin, diclofenac, ibuprofen, Motrin, Midol, naproxen). Others require a prescription (for example, Celebrex). These drugs target the peripheral nervous system and reduce fever and inflammation.

- Acetaminophen or paracetamol (for example, Tylenol, Anacin, Panadol). These drugs appear to act in the central nervous system. Although they reduce fever, they do not reduce inflammation as NSAIDs do.

- Opioids (narcotics). These potent, short-acting (for example, codeine, Dilaudid, Vicodin, Lortab, Percodan, Percocet) and long-acting (for example, methadone, Oxycontin, Duragesic) drugs require a prescription by a physician, dentist, or podiatrist. These drugs target the central nervous system (namely, brain and spinal cord).

NSAIDs have a long history of being prescribed for both acute and chronic pain (Herndon et al., 2008). They have demonstrated short-term benefits for mild to moderate pain (Chou, McDonagh, Nakamoto, & Griffin, 2011); however, they can have significant side effects and should be used only as directed (Bhala et al., 2013; Marsico, Paolillo, & Filardi, 2017).

Acetaminophen or paracetamol is the most commonly used over-the-counter medication for knee osteoarthritis. Although it has been shown to provide benefits in the treatment of mild to moderate pain in patients with osteoarthritis, this has not been observed for patients with back pain (Saragiotto et al., 2016). In general, the results for acetaminophen have been shown to be somewhat less than those seen with NSAIDs and with similar risks of side effects, at least in older patients (Bannuru et al., 2015).

Perhaps the oldest treatment for pain is the use of opioids. Although they have been shown to be effective for short-term use with acute pain (for example, following surgery and trauma) and with patients having pain associated with terminal illnesses, the long-term use for chronic pain has not been demonstrated. For many people, these drugs do not appear to demonstrate significant benefits when used on a long-term basis; moreover, they have been shown to have many negative physical and psychological effects, including significant risks of dependence, misuse, abuse, and addiction (Angarita, Emadi, Hodges, & Morgan, 2016; Ashburn & Fleisher, 2018; Buse et al., 2018; Chou et al., 2015; Furlan, Sandoval, Mailis-Gagnon, & Tunks, 2006). As a consequence, and as we noted in the Introduction, providers are being encouraged and even required to reduce the dosages used and the frequency of prescribing opioids (Dowell, Haegerich, & Chou, 2016). If you have been prescribed opioids, you should discuss your continued use and the dose with your health care prescriber. As with all medications that you have been prescribed, you should not try to change your use on your own. Always discuss your wishes with your health care provider before making any changes.

ANTICONVULSANTS

Anticonvulsant drugs formerly were used only when people had seizures. Now, some anticonvulsants, such as gabapentin (Neurontin), pregabalin (Lyrica), or Topamax (Trileptal) have been shown to have a beneficial effect on pain associated with nerve injuries for some people (for example, those with diabetic neuropathy, trigeminal neuralgia, postherpetic neuralgia). The long-term effects of these new anticonvulsants are unknown because they have not been on the market long enough for such effects to be studied (Wiffen et al., 2013; Zhang et al., 2015). Although it has been hoped that anticonvulsants would have less abuse potential compared with opioids, there have been recent reports of misuse and abuse with gabapentin (Smith, Havens, & Walsh, 2016).

If you are prescribed any of these medications and have found them not to be helpful in a month or so, you should discuss this with your physician and possibly discontinue or change the medication under supervision.

ANTIDEPRESSANTS

Although these drugs are called antidepressants because they were first developed for treating depression, research has shown that they may be helpful in reducing pain. They have effects on neurotransmitters in the brain that affect pain as well as mood. Antidepressants are sometimes effective in relieving pain directly, perhaps due to their effects on serotonin and norepinephrine (neurotransmitters) in the brain. Antidepressants may also help improve sleep. Therefore, they may be used for pain relief even in the absence of depression (Richards, Whittle, & Buchbinder, 2011; Saarto & Wiffen, 2007; Urquhart, Hoving, Assendefft, Roland, & van Tulder, 2008). Antidepressants are sometimes prescribed if the emotions accompanying pain interfere with the ability to function and the quality of life. Some antidepressants help with anxiety and are less likely than antianxiety medications to cause physical dependence when used over an extended period.

Whether to reduce pain directly or help cope with the effects of having a chronic illness, your physician may have prescribed any of the class of drugs labeled as antidepressants (for example, amitriptyline [Elavil], milnacipran [Savella], doxepin [Sinequan], imipramine [Tofranil], trazodone [Desyrel], Prozac, Zoloft). The long-term effects of some of the newest antidepressants are unknown because they have not been on the market long enough for long-term effects to be studied. These are the newest selective serotonin and norepinephrine reuptake inhibitors (SSNRIs), such as venlafaxine (Effexor), duloxetine (Cymbalta), and milnacipran (Savella).

Amitriptyline has been a first-line treatment for neuropathic pain for many years. There is no supportive unbiased evidence for beneficial effects, but that has to be balanced against decades of successful treatment in many people with neuropathic pain. Thus, amitriptyline should probably continue to be used as part of the treatment of neuropathic pain, though only a minority of people will achieve satisfactory pain relief (Moore, Derry, Aldington, Cole, & Wiffen, 2015).

There is some evidence that the newer SSNRI antidepressants can have beneficial effects in reducing pain and improving functioning in patients with osteoarthritis (Wang et al., 2015).

Antidepressant medications usually cause few problems, although they too can cause side effects (namely, nausea, headache, dry mouth, insomnia, constipation, dizziness, fatigue, somnolence, diarrhea, and sweating), with nausea being most common. When the side effects occur, they tend to be mild to moderate, and many resolve over several weeks (Brunton et al., 2010). If you experience side effects that do not remit after a month or so or if your side effects are serious (for example, more than dry mouth or drowsiness or other minor side effects your doctor should tell you about), let your doctor know immediately.

In taking these medications, be aware that they usually take from 2 to 4 weeks before they have an effect. As with any drug, there can also be serious side effects. If you are prescribed an antidepressant and have found it not to be helpful over several months, you should discuss this with your physician and possibly discontinue or change the medication under his or her supervision.

BIOFEEDBACK

Biofeedback is a means of bodily self-monitoring and can be used to help people learn to control certain physiological processes, such as heart rate and muscle tension. For example, under stress, skeletal muscles may contract, causing muscle tension. Biofeedback uses electrical sensors on the skin over muscles to detect this rising tension. The electrical sensors are linked to the biofeedback machine, which provides audible or visual signals to the patient. These signals enable people to understand their physiological activities and to control them consciously and, over time, more automatically. With experience, people can determine what mental or physical adjustments produce the greatest reduction in tension. They may then use these exercises without the need for the biofeedback machine. The greatest amount of research for the benefits of biofeedback has been for headache (Nestoriuc, Martin, Rief, & Andrasik, 2008; Penzien, Irby, Smitherman, Rains, & Houle, 2015), where the benefits appear to be sustained for up to 1 year. Biofeedback has also been used to treat facial pain (for example, temporomandibular joint pain), back pain, and fibromyalgia, among other conditions.

CANNABIS, CANNABINOIDS, AND MARIJUANA

There are a number of components of cannabis, including the compounds cannabidiol (CBD) and tetrahydrocannabinol (THC). To date, the analgesic properties of each are not clear. THC is the psychoactive compound that gives the sensation of euphoria or feeling "high," whereas CBD does not have these effects. There has been growing interest in the medicinal uses of cannabinoids (commonly known as *marijuana* or *weed*, among other terms). Use for pain control is one area where research is currently underway. The results of research on the analgesic benefits of cannabinoids are mixed, and even in those studies showing a benefit, the effects were not substantially higher than achieved with other treatment alternatives (Nugent et al., 2017; Stockings, Campbell, Hall, & Nielsen, 2018).

At the time of this writing, medical and recreational cannabis products are only legal in some states in the United States and a few other countries (for example, Canada). A problem with available products containing cannabinoids is that they are unregulated, and there is little quality control. The potency of the active drug can vary substantially, and the amount of the active components of the drug in any given product are unknown; moreover, the effective dosage can vary widely from person to person. For example, the quantity of cannabinoids in edible products (for example, brownies and gummy candies) is not always clearly labeled. Marijuana cigarettes and vaping pens and cartridges can be of variable sizes, and thus, the quality of the active drug may not be comparable. Thus, although cannabinoids may hold promise as having analgesic properties, more research and quality control measures have to be established. At this point, caution is the most appropriate strategy. You may want to discuss with your physician the use of cannabis as a component of your pain management plan.

COGNITIVE BEHAVIOR THERAPY

Cognitive behavior therapy (CBT) consists of an overriding perspective on people, a set of principles, and a range of techniques to help people learn about themselves and strategies to self-manage their pain and their lives. CBT serves as the guiding set of principles for the approach and strategies included in *The Pain Survival Guide* (Flor & Turk, 2011; Turk, 2018). The key assumptions of the CBT perspective are that

- All people actively process information; they do not merely react to the environment.

- People's thoughts can influence mood and physical arousal, both of which may influence their behavior. Moreover, a person's mood and body state and how they behave can influence their thinking.

- Successful treatments that aim to change problematic (maladaptive) behaviors focus on people's disturbing thoughts and feelings as well as on their behaviors. All are equally important.

- People's behavior is determined by both the external environment and themselves. People do not passively respond to the environment but also prompt (provoke) responses from those around them. Thus, people have a significant influence on others with whom they come in contact.

- Because people develop and maintain problematic (maladaptive) thoughts, feelings, and behaviors, they can change how they think, feel, and behave.

As described throughout this book, there is a range of methods and techniques that can be used to successfully make these changes to your thoughts, feelings, and behaviors. Rather than reacting passively to whatever happens to them or feeling helpless and hopeless, people who use CBT or our CBT-based lessons become more active, resourceful, and resilient. There has been a great deal of research published demonstrating the beneficial effects of CBT with a wide range of pain problems, and some of this is included in Appendix B. It has also been used and shown to be useful for treating people with a number of problematic disorders (for example, eating disorders, depression, posttraumatic stress disorders, sleep disorders, and substance abuse disorders). As a reminder, although the results for CBT have been generally positive, this approach is not a cure but a way to help people cope with and adapt to the challenges that accompany all chronic medical problems, including pain conditions (Ehde, Dillworth, & Turner, 2014; Williams, Eccleston, & Morley, 2012).

EPIDURAL STEROIDS

Epidural steroid injections (ESIs) are a common treatment option for many forms of low back pain and leg pain. They have been used for low back problems since the 1950s and are still an integral part of the nonsurgical management of sciatica and low back pain. The goal of the injection is pain relief; at times, the injection alone is sufficient to provide relief, but commonly, an ESI is used in combination with a comprehensive rehabilitation program to provide additional benefit.

Most practitioners will agree that although the effects of the injection tend to be temporary—providing relief from pain for 1 week up to 1 year—an epidural can be beneficial for a patient during an acute episode of back and/or leg pain. Importantly, an injection can provide sufficient pain relief to allow a patient to progress with a rehabilitative stretching and exercise program. If the initial injection is effective for a patient, he or she may have up to three in 1 year.

Although many studies document the short-term benefits of ESIs, the data on long-term effectiveness are less convincing. Indeed, the effectiveness of lumbar ESIs continues to be a topic of debate (Luijsterburg, Ostelo, Verhagen, & Van Os, 2007; North American Spine Society, 2007; Pinto et al., 2012), and significant risks associated with injection of epidural steroids have been noted (Epstein, 2013).

HYPNOSIS

Hypnosis involves focused attention, reduced peripheral awareness, and an enhanced capacity to respond to suggestion. There are competing theories explaining hypnosis and related phenomena. Altered state theories see hypnosis as an altered state of mind or trance, marked by a level of awareness different from the ordinary state of consciousness. In contrast, nonstate theories see hypnosis as, variously, a type of placebo effect, a redefinition of an interaction with a therapist, or a form of imaginative role enactment. Hypnosis typically incorporates mental imagery and soothing verbal repetition that eases the patient into a trance-like state; once relaxed, patients' minds are more open to transformative messages provided by a therapist. Not everyone is capable of being hypnotized and deriving benefits from hypnotherapy for pain.

Hypnosis has a long history of use in pain management. Positive effects have been reported for the use of hypnosis with a range of acute and chronic pain conditions (Adachi, Fujino, Nkae, Mashimo, & Sasaki, 2014; Jensen & Patterson, 2014), sometimes in combination with other treatments described in this list. If you believe that hypnosis might be something you would like to try, make sure that you seek a provider with the requisite training and skills in work with individuals with chronic pain.

MASSAGE

Massage is the manipulation of soft tissues in the body. Massage techniques are commonly applied with hands, fingers, elbows, knees, forearms, or feet. The purpose of massage is generally for the treatment of body stress or pain.

Several types of massage focus on different parts of the body or healing approaches (for example, deep tissue, Swedish, shiatsu, trigger point), each with some variation. There is no consistent evidence supporting the effectiveness of the various types of message (Furlan, Imamura, Dryden, & Irvin, 2008). During a massage, a massage therapist will apply gentle or strong pressure to the muscles and joints of the body to ease pain and tension. A person who presents himself or herself as a massage therapist should be professionally trained in giving massages.

MINDFULNESS MEDITATION, MINDFULNESS-BASED STRESS REDUCTION, MINDFULNESS-BASED COGNITIVE THERAPY, AND ACCEPTANCE AND COMMITMENT THERAPY

Mindfulness meditation, mindfulness-based stress reduction, mindfulness-based cognitive therapy, and acceptance and commitment therapy are somewhat related and share some of the techniques with CBT, described earlier.

Mindfulness is the psychological process of bringing one's attention to experiences occurring in the present moment, which one can develop through the practice of meditation and other training. Mindfulness and mindfulness meditation focus on becoming aware of all incoming thoughts and feelings and accepting them but not attaching to or reacting to them. Mindfulness can be seen as a strategy that stands in contrast to strategies of avoidance of emotion on the one hand or emotional overengagement on the other hand. Mindfulness can also be viewed as a means to develop self-knowledge and wisdom.

Although some preliminary evidence supports the benefits of mindfulness approaches on some outcomes, there is a need for more research on various mindfulness-based therapies with patients in well-designed and controlled clinical studies for individuals with different chronic pain disorders (Hilton et al., 2017; Hughes, Clark, Colclough, Dale, & McMillan, 2017; Reiner, Tibi, & Lipsitz, 2013; Veehof, Trompetter, Bohlmeijer, & Schreurs, 2016).

MIXED AGENT DRUGS

There is one medication frequently prescribed for pain that does not exactly fit in any of the other categories—tramadol (Ultram). At high doses, tramadol has some of the properties of opioids and at low doses appears to act more like an antidepressant. Tramadol has side effects that are similar to opioids, including risks for abuse (Babalonis, Lofwall, Nuzzo, Siegel, & Walsh, 2013; Bush, 2015). If you are taking this prescribed medication for your pain, be sure to discuss the risks with your physician.

NERVE BLOCKS

Local anesthetic agents (for example, lidocaine) that are similar to Novocain may be injected into peripheral nerve fibers when the physician believes the pain is being generated, transferred, or referred. The most common form of this procedure is called an *epidural block*. Here, a local anesthetic is injected between the vertebrae into spinal nerves. Many other nerves can also be "blocked" by injecting the anesthetic into them. Injection of steroids into the epidural space surrounding the spinal cord and nerves may be helpful in sciatica (leg pain secondary to disc disease). These injections will cause the nerve fibers to become numb (anesthetized). Specially trained physicians, usually anesthesiologists, are qualified to perform nerve blocks. Some people feel immediate reductions of pain following these injections. Others do not feel any relief. The duration of relief, when obtained, varies unpredictably from hours to days to weeks. However, the effects do not appear to last indefinitely for anyone. The available results on the long-term benefits are mixed (Merrill, 2003; Turk, Wilson, & Cahana, 2011; Wasan et al., 2009).

PAIN CLINICS AND REHABILITATION PROGRAMS

Specialized pain clinics and rehabilitation programs have been developed over the past 30 years to treat people with chronic pain. These programs usually use many of the techniques described in this book and this appendix, most often in combination. In addition to including physicians on their staff, the best programs have psychologists who can teach stress management and coping skills. They can also help people improve their communication with family members and health care professionals. Most clinics also have physical and occupational therapists on staff to help people learn new ways to improve their strength, endurance, and functioning while they perform household and on-the-job tasks.

Comprehensive programs have been shown to be quite effective for helping many people with severe, long-standing pain problems reduce their pain and emotional distress and improve physical functioning in the short term; however, long-term effects are more mixed (Kamper et al., 2014). You should discuss the appropriateness of a referral to a pain clinic with your primary care doctor. If your doctor is unfamiliar with such clinics, seek out a doctor who is familiar with them (but is not on their staff) and ask whether he or she thinks it is worth your while to try such a program.

PHYSICAL THERAPY AND OCCUPATIONAL THERAPY

The general class of physical and occupational therapies includes a wide range of treatments. These may consist of a variety of strengthening, conditioning, and flexibility exercises that are supervised by a physical therapist, occupational therapist, or exercise physiologist. These exercises are often used in combination with other treatments for chronic pain—for example, ultrasound (described earlier) and diathermy (see "Thermal Therapies"). Although frequently recommended, there is no evidence that any particular form of exercise provides greater benefits than any other (Hayden, van Tulder, Malmivara, & Koes, 2005; Ross & Thomas, 2010), although aerobic exercises appear to provide the greatest benefit compared with strengthening and flexibility exercises for patients with fibromyalgia (Busch, Barber, Overend, Peloso, & Schachter, 2007).

PILATES

Pilates is a physical fitness system developed in the early 20th century by Joseph Pilates, after whom it was named. Pilates exercises are designed to improve flexibility, build strength, and develop control and endurance in the entire body. This system emphasizes alignment, breathing, developing a strong core, and improving coordination and balance. It incorporates breathing, concentration, control, centering, flow, postural alignment, precision, relaxation, and stamina. Body core exercises focus on the muscles of the abdomen, low back, and hips.

There is only limited evidence to support the use of Pilates to alleviate low back pain or improve balance in older people (Wells, Kolt, Marshall, Hill, & Bialocerkowski, 2014). Evidence from studies shows that although Pilates improves balance, limited data exist on whether this impacts the number of falls for older adults. Pilates has not been shown to be an effective treatment for any specific medical condition. There is some evidence that regular Pilates sessions can help muscle conditioning in healthy adults, compared with doing no exercise.

SEDATIVES, TRANQUILIZERS, AND MUSCLE RELAXANTS

Sedatives and minor tranquilizers (for example, benzodiazepines)—such as diazepam (Valium), lorazepam (Ativan), and clonazepam (Klonopin)—and muscle relaxants (for example, cyclobenzaprine [Flexeril] and methocarbamol [Robaxin]) may be prescribed to help people cope with anxiety and also improve their sleep (Abdel Shaheed et al., 2017; Cheatle & Shmuts, 2015). These may be used in combination with analgesics. Sedatives, tranquilizers, and muscle relaxants may help relieve short-term anxiety about pain. They also have more immediate effects than antidepressants. However, they are not appropriate for long-term use for people with chronic pain because of their definite potential for addiction when used on a long-term basis (more than a few months; Gauntlett-Gilbert, Gavriloff, & Brook, 2016). Again, if you are prescribed any of these medications and have found them not to be helpful after several weeks, you should discuss this with your physician and possibly discontinue or change the medication, under supervision.

SPINAL CORD STIMULATION

Spinal cord stimulation (SCS) or dorsal column stimulation is a type of implantable neuromodulation device that is used to send electrical signals to select areas of the spinal cord for the treatment of certain pain conditions. SCS is a costly, invasive procedure that should be considered only for people whose pain condition has not responded to more conservative therapy. The most common indications for SCS include failed back surgery syndrome, peripheral neuropathy of any etiology, chronic regional pain syndrome, phantom pain, facial neuropathy, radiculitis, and postherpetic neuralgia. The effectiveness of SCS remains quite controversial. It may have some benefits for carefully selected patients (Kumar et al., 2006; Rosenow et al., 2006; Turner, Hollingworth, Comstock, & Deyo, 2010).

SPINAL MANIPULATIONS (CHIROPRACTIC, OSTEOPATHIC, MANUAL THERAPY)

In chiropractic and osteopathic theory, muscle and joint pain are thought to result from faulty relationships among bones and faulty alignment of the spine. Chiropractors perform manipulations—often quite strenuously—to return the bones or spinal cord to "proper" alignment. Sometimes these are quite helpful, particularly in the early stages of an injury, such as whiplash. However, over a long period, they may become less effective (Rubinstein et al., 2019).

SURGERY

Surgery is appropriate with certain kinds of pathology causing acute pain. There are a large variety of surgical approaches that can help, depending on the pathology that is believed to be the "pain generator." However, when pain persists over long periods, surgery is less likely to be effective. Also, if you have already had one operation, it is unlikely that more surgery will eliminate the pain (Franklin, Haug, Heyer, McKeefrey, & Picciano, 1994). A second operation may, however, be justified if the initial cause of your pain has progressed as part of a degenerative disease or your physical condition has deteriorated.

When surgery is being considered, you should discuss this with your primary physician and a qualified surgeon. Obtaining a second surgical opinion is recommended because surgeons differ in their approach to surgery as well. A second opinion also has the benefit of helping you judge which surgeon is more qualified to conduct the surgery. Because surgery has the potential for ill as well as good, do your homework and be well informed before you elect to undergo surgery or choose a surgeon.

TAI CHI AND YOGA

There are many other types of exercise systems used in treating people with chronic pain in addition to the ones described in this section.

Tai chi is an ancient Chinese tradition that, today, is practiced as a graceful form of exercise. It involves a series of movements performed in a slow, focused manner and accompanied by deep breathing. Tai chi is a self-paced system of gentle physical exercise and stretching. Each posture flows into the next without pause, ensuring that your body is in constant motion.

Tai chi has many different styles. Each style may subtly emphasize various tai chi principles and methods. There are variations within each style. Some styles may focus on health maintenance, whereas others focus on the martial arts aspect of tai chi. Tai chi is different from yoga, another type of meditative movement. Although tai chi has been shown to have some short-term beneficial effects for individuals with chronic back pain (Hall, Maher, Lam, Ferreira, & Latimer, 2011), no evidence has been reporting suggesting that any one style is significantly more effective than any other.

Yoga is a group of physical, mental, and spiritual practices or disciplines that originated in ancient India. Yoga includes various physical postures and breathing techniques, along with meditation. The term *yoga* in the Western world often includes the physical practice of postures. There are a number of approaches to yoga emphasizing different sets of postures and different levels of speed and intensity. As with tai chi, although yoga can provide some beneficial effects for people with chronic pain, there is no support for any one type compared with any other (Cramer, Lauche, Haller, & Dubos, 2013).

Postural yoga has been studied and may be recommended to promote relaxation, reduce stress, and improve some medical conditions, such as chronic back pain. Yoga is considered to be a low-impact activity that can provide the same benefits as any well-designed exercise program, increasing general health and stamina, reducing stress, and improving those conditions brought about by sedentary lifestyles. It is particularly promoted as a physical therapy routine and as a regimen to strengthen and balance all parts of the body.

The American College of Sports Medicine cites yoga's "promotion of profound mental, physical and spiritual awareness" and its benefits as a form of stretching and as an enhancer of breath control and core strength.

THERMAL THERAPIES

Both heat and cold therapy can reduce muscle tension (French, Cameron, Walker, Reggars, & Esterman, 2006). Heat can reduce muscle contractions (spasms) caused by overfatigue of muscles. Applying heat to sore, fatigued muscles tends to open (therefore, dilate) blood vessels and thus increases oxygen flow and eliminates chemical irritants. Cold can also reduce muscle spasms and swelling from an injury or inflammation. Heat and cold have been found to be about equally effective and may be used separately or together (namely one following the other; French et al., 2006). They are useful home remedies that are also used during and after physical therapy sessions (Brosseau et al., 2003). Many have found that frozen peas in a bag wrapped in a towel are more useful and convenient than ice packs. They can be "molded" around a painful body part, such as the forearm. They can be refrozen and used over and over again (be sure not to eat them afterward, however).

TOPICAL AGENTS

Several topical agents, such as Zostrix, 5% lidocaine patch (Lidoderm), 8% capsaicin (Quienza), topical NSAIDs (for example, diclofenac and ketoprofen) have been shown to reduce the severity of pain in some conditions related to nerve damage. In some studies, these agents have been shown to have a positive effect with short-term use (for example, Galer, Rowbotham, Perander, & Friedman, 1999). There is limited evidence for the benefits for long-term use (Derry, Wiffen, Moore, & Guinlan, 2014; Jones, Moore, & Peterson, 2011; McPherson & Cimino, 2013). Although these topical agents have been reported to provide good relief for patients with osteoarthritis, the results are not much greater than seen with nonactive agents (placebos) in randomized controlled trials (Derry, Conaghan, Da Silva, Wiffen, & Moore, 2016).

There are a number of other topical agents available from pharmacies that do not require prescriptions. There is little evidence of the benefits of the non-prescription topical agents. If you are prescribed any of these medications and have found them not to be helpful after several weeks, you should discuss this with your physician and possibly discontinue or change the medication under supervision.

TRANSCUTANEOUS ELECTRIC NERVE STIMULATION

Transcutaneous electrical nerve stimulation (TENS) is the use of electric current produced by a device to stimulate the nerves for therapeutic purposes. TENS, by definition, covers the complete range of transcutaneously applied currents used for nerve excitation, although the term is often used with a more restrictive intent—namely, to describe the kind of pulses produced by portable stimulators used to treat pain. The unit is usually connected to the skin using two or more electrodes. A typical battery-operated TENS unit can modulate pulse width, frequency, and intensity.

TENS is generally applied at high frequency with an intensity below motor contraction or low frequency with an intensity that produces a motor contraction. Although the use of TENS has proved effective in some clinical studies, there is a lack of consensus as to as which conditions the device should be used to treat (Buchmuller et al., 2012).

TRIGGER POINT INJECTIONS

Trigger points are hypersensitive areas of muscles, ligaments, or tendons. They are known to lie above or near the point in the muscles where the motor nerves are located. Excessive activity in motor nerves can produce pain either at the site or at some other site—this is known as *referred pain*. There are standard patterns of referred pain associated with specific injuries. When these trigger points are pressed, it can cause a great deal of pain.

Direct stress to the muscle, as in trauma (for example, a muscle tear during a motor vehicle accident or a tendon inflamed during repetitive activity), chronic tension, abnormal posture, or prolonged muscle fatigue may result in pain in these trigger point areas.

This is relevant to chronic pain because some who experience chronic pain tend to tense their muscles in an attempt to brace and therefore protect themselves from pain. This, in turn, can lead to the pain–muscle spasm–pain circle. When in spasm, muscles tend to remain in a tense or contracted state, blood flow is decreased to the muscle, and posture can become abnormal. This may serve to maintain the pain or make it worse. Also, some trigger points may become inactive from sedentary living, which is unfortunately common in many chronic pain patients. Trigger-point pain can then be reactivated by minor stress from daily living, anxiety, overstretching, or sudden use, overuse, and fatigue of previously underworked muscles.

Trigger point injections are a relatively safe procedure when used by clinicians with appropriate expertise and training. A variety of different agents may be injected at specific tender points, most commonly local anesthetics or combinations of these agents (for example, Novocain, lidocaine), corticosteroids, or combinations of anesthetic agents and corticosteroids. As with many of the treatments described for chronic pain management, there is no clear evidence for the benefits of trigger point injections (Scott, Guo, Barton, & Gerwin, 2009).

ULTRASOUND STIMULATION

Ultrasound, either with heat (in fatty areas) or without heat (in bony areas) has also been found to be useful for low back pain, particularly in cases of acute musculoskeletal injury leading to chronic pain (DeSantana, Walsh, Vance, Rakel, & Saluka, 2008; Ebadi et al., 2014).

APPENDIX B

Additional Reading

Many of the books listed here are available for purchase on the Internet or can be checked out at local libraries.

LESSON 1: BECOMING YOUR OWN PAIN MANAGEMENT EXPERT

Caudill, M. A. (2009). *Managing pain before it manages you* (3rd ed.). New York, NY: Guilford Press.
Croft, P., Blyth, F. M., & van der Windt, D. (2010). *Chronic pain epidemiology: From aetiology to public health.* New York, NY: Oxford University Press.
Institute of Medicine. (2011). *Relieving pain in America: A blueprint for transforming prevention, care, education, and research.* Washington, DC: National Academies Press.
Melzack, R., & Wall, P. D. (1982). *The challenge of pain.* New York, NY: Basic Books.

LESSON 2: ACTIVITY, REST, AND PACING

Allen, D. (2015). *Getting things done: The art of stress-free productivity* (2nd ed.). New York, NY: Penguin.
Christy, C., Cheever, R., Garee, B., & Sarafconn, C. A. (1990). *Pacing yourself: Steps to helping save your energy.* Bloomington, IL: Cheever.
Gates, R., & Kenison, K. (2002). *Meditations from the mat: Daily reflections on the path of yoga.* New York, NY: Random House.
Iknoian, T. (2005). *Fitness walking* (2nd ed.). Champaign, IL: Human Kinetics.
Inkeles G., & Schencke, I. (1994). *Ergonomic living: How to create a user-friendly home and office.* New York, NY: Simon & Schuster.
Matthews, J. (2016). *Stretching to stay young: Simple workouts to keep you flexible, energized, and pain free.* Berkeley, CA: Althea Press.
Ornstein, R., & Sobel, D. (1989). *Healthy pleasures.* Reading, MA: Addison Wesley.
Reynolds, D. K. (2002). *A handbook for constructive living.* Honolulu: University of Hawaii Press.
Ryan, M. J. (2003). *The power of patience.* New York, NY: Random House.
Schaef, A. W. (2004). *Meditations for women who do too much* (rev. ed.). San Francisco, CA: HarperOne. [Available for Kindle]

Wilson, A. (1994). *Are you sitting comfortably? A self-help guide for sufferers of back pain, neck strain, headaches, RSI, and other health problems.* London, England: Optima.

LESSON 3: LEARNING TO RELAX

Achtenberg, J., Dossey, B., & Kolkneier, L. (1994). *Rituals of healing: Using imagery for health and wellness.* New York, NY: Bantam Books.

Benson, H. (2000). *The relaxation response* (rev. ed.). New York, NY: HarperCollins.

Bernstein, D. A., Borkovec, T. D., & Hazlett-Stevens, H. (2000). *New directions in progressive relaxation training: A guidebook for the helping professions.* Westport, CT: Praeger.

Borysenko, J. M. (2007). *Minding the body, mending the mind.* New York, NY: Da Capo Press.

Casey, K. (2001). *Each day a new beginning: A meditation book and journal for self-reflection.* Center City, MN: Hazelden.

Davis, M., Eshelman, E. R., & McKay, M. (2000). *The relaxation and stress reduction workbook.* Oakland, CA: New Harbinger.

Fanning, P. (1994). *Visualization for change* (2nd ed.). Oakland, CA: New Harbinger.

Kabat-Zinn, J. (2007). *Arriving at your own door: 108 lessons in mindfulness.* New York, NY: Hyperion.

Kabat-Zinn, J. (2013). *Full catastrophe living: Using the wisdom of your body and mind to face stress, pain, and illness* (rev. ed.). New York, NY: Random House.

Ruhnke, A., & Wurzburger, A. (1995). *Body wisdom: Simple massage and relaxation techniques for busy people.* Boston, MA: Charles Tuttle.

Weintraub, A. (2004). *Yoga for depression: A compassionate guide to relieve suffering through yoga.* New York, NY: Random House.

Young, S. (1995). *Break through pain: How to relieve pain using powerful meditation techniques* [Audiotape]. Louisville, CO: Sounds True.

Young, S. (2004). *Pain relief* [CD]. Louisville, CO: Sounds True.

LESSON 4: ARE YOU ALWAYS TIRED? WAYS TO COMBAT FATIGUE

American Heart Association. (2004). *American Heart Association low-fat, low cholesterol cook book: Delicious recipes to help lower your cholesterol* (3rd ed.). New York, NY: Clarkson Potter.

Ancoli-Israel, S. (1996). *All I want is a good night's sleep.* St. Louis, MO: Mosby.

Barsky, A., & Deans, E. C. (2006). *Feeling better: A 6-week mind–body program to ease your chronic symptoms.* New York, NY: HarperCollins.

Catalano, E. M. (1990). *Getting to sleep.* Oakland, CA: New Harbinger.

Hauri, P., & Linde, S. (1991). *No more sleepless nights.* New York, NY: Wiley.

Jacobs, G. (1998). *Say goodnight to insomnia: The six-week, drug-free program developed at Harvard Medical School.* New York, NY: Holt.

Willett, W. C., & Skerrett, P. J. (2005). *Eat, drink, and be healthy: The Harvard Medical School guide to healthy eating.* New York, NY: Free Press.

LESSON 5: DON'T LET PAIN RUIN YOUR RELATIONSHIPS!

Bower, S. A., & Bower, G. H. (2004). *Asserting yourself.* Reading, MA: Addison-Wesley.

Duck, S. W., & McMahan, D. T. (2010). *Communication in everyday life*. Thousand Oaks, CA: SAGE.

Engel, B. (2004). *Honor your anger: How transforming your anger style can change your life*. Hoboken, NJ: Wiley.

Gentry, W. D. (2007). *Anger management for dummies*. Hoboken, NJ: Wiley.

Hendrix, H., & Hunt, H. L. (2004). *Receiving love: Transform your relationship by letting yourself be loved*. New York, NY: Atria Books.

Jakubowski, P. (1978). *The assertive option*. Champaign, IL: Research Press.

Kahane, A., & Senge, P. M. (2007). *Solving tough problems: An open way of talking, listening, and creating new realities*. San Francisco, CA: Berrett-Koehler.

McKay, M., Davis, M., & Fanning, P. (1995). *Messages: The communication skills book* (2nd ed.). Oakland, CA: New Harbinger.

Pennebaker, J. W., & Evans, J. F. (2014). *Expressive writing: Words that heal*. Enumclaw, WA: Idyll Arbor.

Tannen, D. (1986). *That's not what I meant! How conversational style makes or breaks relationships*. New York, NY: Ballantine Books.

Tannen, D. (2001). *You just don't understand: Women and men in conversation*. New York, NY: Harper Paperbacks.

LESSON 6: CHANGING BEHAVIOR

Armstrong L., & Jenkins, S. (2000). *It's not about the bike*. New York, NY: Berkley.

Bridges, W. (2003). *Managing transitions: Making the most of change*. Cambridge, MA: Perseus.

Ilardo, J., & Rothman, C. (2003). *Take a chance: Risks to grow by*. New York, NY: MJF Books.

McKay, M., Davis, M., & Fanning P. (2011). *Thoughts and feelings* (4th ed.). Richmond, CA: New Harbinger.

Nicholas, M., Molloy, A., Tonkin, L., & Beeston, L. (2000). *Manage your pain*. Sydney, Australia: ABC Books.

Price, R. (1994). *A whole new life*. New York, NY: Atheneum.

LESSON 7: CHANGING THOUGHTS AND FEELINGS

Burns, D. (1999). *The feeling good handbook* (2nd ed.). New York, NY: William Morrow.

Ellis, A. (1999). *How to make yourself happy and remarkably less disturbable*. Manassas Park, VA: Impact.

Greenberger, D., & Padesky, C. A. (2016). *Mind over mood: A cognitive therapy treatment manual for clients* (2nd ed.). New York, NY: Guilford Press.

Seligman, M. (2006). *Learned optimism: How to change your mind and your life*. New York, NY: Vintage Books.

LESSON 8: GAINING SELF-CONFIDENCE

D'Zurilla, T. J., & Nezu, A. M. (2007). *Problem solving therapy: A positive approach to clinical intervention* (3rd ed.). New York, NY: Springer.

Hoenig, C. W. (2000). *The problem solving journey: Your guide to making decisions and getting results*. Reading, VA: Basic Books.

McKay, M., & Fanning, P. (2000). *Self-esteem: A proven program of cognitive techniques for assessing, improving, and maintaining your self-esteem.* Oakland, CA: New Harbinger.

Nezu, A. M., Nezu, C. M., & D'Zurilla, T. J. (2012). *Problem-solving therapy: A treatment manual.* New York, NY: Springer.

Taylor, S. (1999). *Living well with a hidden disability: Transcending doubt and shame and reclaiming your life.* Oakland, CA: New Harbinger.

LESSON 9: PUTTING IT ALL TOGETHER

Alberti, R. E., & Emmons, M. I. (2008). *Your perfect right: A guide to assertive living* (9th ed.). Atascadero, CA: Impact.

Allen, J. (2006). *As a man thinketh.* Los Angeles, CA: Penguin Putnam Press.

Brach, T. (2003). *Radical self-acceptance.* New York, NY: Bantam.

Cloud, H. (2003). *Changes that heal.* Grand Rapids, MI: Zondervan.

LESSON 10: MAINTENANCE AND COPING WITH SETBACKS

Benson, H., & Stuart, E. (1993). *The wellness book: The comprehensive guide to maintaining health and treating stress-related illness.* Secaucus, NJ: Birch Lane Press.

Marlatt, G. A., & Gordon, J. R. (2005). *Relapse prevention: A self-control strategy for the maintenance of behavior change* (2nd ed.). New York, NY: Guilford Press.

Web and Mobile Resources for Pain

In this appendix, we list only a few of the available websites, health news outlets, blogs, podcasts, social media sites, and apps you can explore as you design your pain self-management program. In addition to the resources listed here, there are many more. We do not endorse or attest to the accuracy of the information included in any of these. Our intent is to alert you to some of the many available resources.

We advise caution when using any health apps because the legal standards that apply to your medical records do not necessarily apply to apps. If your health insurer or health care provider's office offers an app that connects to your medical record, this is more likely to be covered by patient privacy laws. Recommendations for using health apps safely are available at such outlets as *Consumer Reports*, *Wired*, and *CNET*. In addition, the article by Zhao, Yoo, Lancey, and Varghese (2019) contains a review of pain-relevant health applications available and some of their limitations.

GENERAL

American Chronic Pain Association

http://www.theacpa.org

The American Chronic Pain Association (ACPA) has been helping people with chronic illness for the past 35 years. This website offers an A to Z guide to various pain conditions, a comprehensive prescription and over-the-counter drug list, relaxation videos, a "coping calendar" with daily coping ideas and activities, resources to help you work more collaboratively with your health team, and a shop where you can purchase literature and CDs. ACPA has a large number of self-help group affiliates across the United States and Canada.

American Geriatrics Society

http://www.americangeriatrics.org; http://www.healthinaging.org

This site is geared toward health care professionals who work with older adults. Its resources include clinical guidelines for the management of persistent pain in older adults. For the general public, the American Geriatrics Society offers the Health in Aging site, which includes resources for caregivers, a searchable directory of health care providers who specialize in the care of older adults, and a blog (use the Search function to find articles about pain or other topics).

U.S. Pain Foundation, Pain Connection, Ouchie App

http://www.uspainfoundation.org; http://www.PainConnection.org

Pain Connection offers support in the form of in-person groups, telephone conferences, and a specialized therapy group for military veterans. There are also online-only support groups for specific conditions such as rheumatoid arthritis, fibromyalgia, endometriosis, and multiple sclerosis. The U.S. Pain Foundation also has an app called Ouchie, developed with input from pain sufferers and health care professionals that allows users to educate themselves about their condition and latest developments in pain management, track their pain, and share experiences with others (sharing and privacy settings can be adjusted).

Positivity in Pain

https://www.facebook.com/PositiveInPain/

A support group created by author Jennifer Corter, providing videos, articles, and user-created content to help users interact and laugh along with others living with similar conditions.

Healthtalk

http://www.healthtalk.org

Features first-person videos by teens and adults of all ages with various health conditions, including chronic pain. All content is based on qualitative research into patients' experiences of health conditions. The site is a partnership between a United Kingdom-based charity called DIPEx International and The Health Experiences Research Group at Oxford University's Nuffield Department of Primary Care Health Sciences.

Pain Concern, Airing Pain Podcast

http://www.painconcern.org.uk

Provides support for those with pain and their caregivers and has fact sheets and videos on different aspects of chronic pain and self-management. It also contains links to listen and subscribe to Airing Pain, a free podcast series on living with pain.

Relief: Pain Research News, Insights, and Ideas

http://www.relief.news
   News source sponsored by the International Association for the Study of Pain.

ARTHRITIS

Arthritis Foundation

http://www.arthritis.org
   Along with self-care tips, such as anti-inflammatory diet ideas, this site includes a finder function to help users locate local arthritis resources such as community events, fundraisers, health care providers, fitness programs and coaching, home health care providers, and medical equipment suppliers. It also includes an Educational Rights Toolkit for children with arthritis.

BACK PAIN

Spine Universe

http://www.Spineuniverse.com
   This is a health news site specifically for people with lower back and general back pain. It includes an online community feature for sharing advice with others who have back pain; a specialist locator feature for the United States, Canada, and other countries; information on clinical trials; and a video library of helpful exercises for back health.

ENDOMETRIOSIS

Endometriosis UK

http://www.endometriosis-uk.org
   This charity provides information and support for women and teen girls with endometriosis, including diagnosis, treatment, fertility issues, and advice for couples on intimacy and coping.

FIBROMYALGIA

National Fibromyalgia and Chronic Pain Association

http://www.fibroandpain.org
   This site offers a support group search function, an online forum, articles about fibromyalgia, and a directory of health care providers. It also includes calls to action for people with fibromyalgia who wish to contribute to advocacy efforts such as advising policy makers about their experiences.

HEADACHE

American Migraine Foundation

http://www.americanmigrainefoundation.org

This site offers downloadable patient guides with tips for communicating with your employer about your headaches, meal planning, applying for Social Security Disability, and coping with migraine during holidays, among other topics. It also features links to get involved in advocacy. The organization has active Facebook and Instagram communities, as well.

National Headache Foundation, Heads Up Podcast

http://www.headaches.org

In addition to its publication library and provider search function, this website offers a clinical trial match function, links to a podcast called Heads Up, and a special set of resources for college students coping with headaches. It also offers how-to worksheets for navigating insurance issues and caring for a loved one with migraines.

Migraine Monitor App

http://www.migrainemonitor.com

The app allows users to track headaches, their severity, duration, and triggers and provides access to health care professionals as well as an anonymous community of other headache sufferers. It also generates reports and provides a daily information feed. The app was designed by neurologists and is recommended by the National Headache Foundation.

N1-Headache App

http://www.n1-headache.com

The N1-Headache app allows users to "test" behavioral changes that may reduce the number or severity of their attacks. The app generates a personal analytical report that users can share with their clinician.

PELVIC PAIN

International Pelvic Pain Society, Women's Pelvic Health Podcast

http://www.pelvicpain.org/IPPS/patients

The patient-focused portion of this site includes a provider search function, pamphlets on specific pelvic conditions, a store site to purchase vaginal dilators, and links to listen and subscribe to podcasts about pelvic pain.

Pelvic Pain Support Network

http://www.pelvicpain.org.uk

The Pelvic Pain Support Network provides information on pelvic pain conditions and tips for how to talk with providers, family and friends, and employers about pelvic pain, plus a message forum for members where they can find support and ask the advice of other members of the public. Conditions covered include endometriosis, vulvar pain, Crohn's Disease, and interstitial cystitis.

Research Supporting This Pain Management Program

GENERAL

Buhrman, M., Fredriksson, A., Edstrom, G., Shafiei, D., Tärnqvist, C., Ljótsson, B., . . . Andersson, G. (2013). Guided internet-delivered cognitive behavioural therapy for chronic pain patients who have residual symptoms after rehabilitation treatment: Randomized controlled trial. *European Journal of Pain, 17*, 753–765. http://dx.doi.org/10.1002/j.1532-2149.2012.00244.x

Deary, V., Chalder, T., & Sharpe, M. (2007). The cognitive behavioural model of medically unexplained symptoms: A theoretical and empirical review. *Clinical Psychology Review, 27*, 781–797. http://dx.doi.org/10.1016/j.cpr.2007.07.002

Ehde, D. H., Dillworth, T. M., & Turner, J. A. (2014). Cognitive-behavioral therapy for individuals with chronic pain: Efficacy, innovations, and directions for research. *American Psychologist, 69*, 153–166. http://dx.doi.org/10.1037/a0035747

Okifuji, A., & Turk, D. C. (2015). Behavioral and cognitive–behavioral approaches to treating patients with chronic pain: Thinking outside the pill box. *Journal of Rational-Emotive and Cognitive-Behavior Therapy, 33*, 218–238. http://dx.doi.org/10.1007/s10942-015-0215-x

Skinner, M., Wilson, H. D., & Turk, D. C. (2012). Cognitive-behavioral perspective and cognitive-behavioral therapy for people with chronic pain: Distinctions, outcomes, and innovations. *Journal of Cognitive Psychotherapy, 26*, 93–113. http://dx.doi.org/10.1891/0889-8391.26.2.93

Thorn, B. E. (2004). *Cognitive therapy for chronic pain: A step-by-step guide.* New York, NY: Guilford Press.

Turk, D. C., & Gatchel, R. J. (Eds.). (2018). *Psychological approaches to pain management: A practitioner's handbook* (3rd ed.). New York, NY: Guilford Press.

Williams, A. C. de C., Eccleston, C., & Morley, S. (2012). Psychological therapies for the management of chronic pain (excluding headache) in adults. *Cochrane Database of Systematic Reviews, 11*, CD007407. http://dx.doi.org/10.1002/14651858. CD007407.pub3

ARTHRITIS

Broderick, J. E., Keefe, F. J., Bruckenthal, P., Junghaenel, D. U., Schneider, S., Schwartz, J. E., . . . Gould, E. (2014). Nurse practitioners can effectively deliver pain coping skills training to osteoarthritis patients with chronic pain: A randomized, controlled trial. *Pain, 155*, 1743–1754. http://dx.doi.org/10.1016/j.pain.2014.05.024

Hunt, M. A., Keefe, F. J., Bryant, C., Metcalf, B. R., Ahamed, Y., Nicholas, M. K., & Bennell, K. L. (2013). A physiotherapist-delivered, combined exercise and pain coping skills training intervention for individuals with knee osteoarthritis: A pilot study. *Knee, 20*, 106–112. http://dx.doi.org/10.1016/j.knee.2012.07.008

Sharpe, L., Sensky, T., Timberlake, N., Ryan, B., Brewin, C. R., & Allard, S. (2001). A blind, randomized, controlled trial of cognitive-behavioural intervention for patients with recent onset rheumatoid arthritis: Preventing psychological and physical morbidity. *Pain, 89*, 275–283. http://dx.doi.org/10.1016/S0304-3959(00)00379-1

BACK PAIN

Cherkin, D. C., Sherman, K. J, Balderson, B. H., Cook, A. J., Anderson, M. L., Hawkes, R. J., . . . Turner, J. A. (2016). Effect of mindfulness-based stress reduction vs cognitive behavioral therapy or usual care on back pain and functional limitations in adults with chronic low back pain: A randomized clinical trial. *JAMA, 315*, 1240–1249. http://dx.doi.org/10.1001/jama.2016.2323

Henschke, N., Ostelo, R. W. J. G., van Tulder, M. W., Vlaeyen, J. W. S., Morley, S., Assendelft, W. J. J., & Main, C. J. (2010), Behavioral treatment for chronic low-back pain. *Cochrane Database of Systematic Reviews, 7*, CD002014. http://dx.doi.org/10.1002/14651858.CD002014.pub3

Lamb, S. E., Hansen, Z., Lall, R., Castelnuovo, E., Withers, E. J., Nichols, V., . . . Back Skills Training Trial investigators. (2010). Group cognitive behavioural treatment for low-back pain in primary care: A randomised controlled trial and cost-effectiveness analysis. *The Lancet, 375*, 916–923. http://dx.doi.org/10.1016/S0140-6736(09)62164-4

Linton, S. J., Boersma, K., Traczyk, M., Shaw, W., & Nicholas, M. (2016). Early workplace communication and problem solving to prevent back disability: Results of a randomized controlled trial among high-risk workers and their supervisors. *Journal of Occupational Rehabilitation, 26*, 150–159. http://dx.doi.org/10.1007/s10926-015-9596-z

Linton, S. J., & Nordin, E. (2006). A 5-year follow-up evaluation of the health and economic consequences of an early cognitive behavioral intervention for back pain: A randomized, controlled trial. *Spine, 31*, 853–858. http://dx.doi.org/10.1097/01.brs.0000209258.42037.02

Richmond, H., Hall, A. M., Copsey, B., Hansen, Z., Williamson, E., Hoxey-Thomas, N., . . . Lamb, S. E. (2015). The effectiveness of cognitive behavioural treatment for non-specific low back pain: A systematic review and meta-analysis. *PLOS One, 10*, e0134192. http://dx.doi.org/10.1371/journal.pone.0134192

Turner, J. A., Anderson, M. L., Balderson, B. H., Cook, A. J., Sherman, K. J., & Cherkin, D. C. (2016). Mindfulness-based stress reduction and cognitive behavioral therapy for chronic low back pain: Similar effects on mindfulness, catastrophizing, self-efficacy, and acceptance in a randomized controlled trial. *Pain, 157*, 2434–2444. http://dx.doi.org/10.1097/j.pain.0000000000000635

CANCER-RELATED PAIN

Dalton, J. A., Keefe, F. J., Carlson, J., & Youngblood, R. (2004). Tailoring cognitive-behavioral treatment for cancer pain. *Pain Management Nursing, 5*, 3–18. http://dx.doi.org/10.1016/s1524-9042(03)00027-4

Kwekkeboom, K. L., Cherwin, C. H., Lee, J. W., & Wanta, B. (2010). Mind-body treatments for pain-fatigue-sleep disturbance symptom clusters in person with cancer. *Journal of Pain and Symptom Management, 39*, 126–138. http://dx.doi.org/10.1016/j.jpainsymman.2009.05.022

Sheinfeld Gorin, S., Krebs, P., Badr, H., Janke, E. A., Jim, H. S., Spring, B., . . . Jacobsen, P. B. (2012). Meta-analysis of psychosocial interventions to reduce pain in patients with cancer. *Journal of Clinical Oncology, 30*, 539–547. http://dx.doi.org/10.1200/JCO.2011.37.0437

Syrjala, K. L., Jensen, M. P., Mendoza, M. E., Yi, J. C., Fisher, H. M., & Keefe, F. J. (2014). Psychological and behavioral approaches to cancer pain management. *Journal of Clinical Oncology, 32*, 1703–1711. http://dx.doi.org/10.1200/JCO.2013.54.4825

CHILDREN AND ADOLESCENTS WITH CHRONIC PAIN

(Although not the focus of this book, we include references for those who might be interested in the potential use of this program with children and adolescents.)

Eccleston, C., Palermo, T. M., Williams, A. C. de C., Holley, A. L., Morley, S., Fisher, E., & Law, E. (2014). Psychological therapies for the management of chronic and recurrent pain in children and adolescents. *Cochrane Database of Systematic Reviews, 5*, CD003968. http://dx.doi.org/10.1002/14651858.CD003968.pub4

Fisher, E., Heathcote, L., Palermo, T. M., Williams, A. C. de C., Lau, J., & Eccleston, C. (2014). Systematic review and meta-analysis of psychological therapies for children with chronic pain. *Journal of Pediatric Psychology, 39*, 763–782. http://dx.doi.org/10.1093/jpepsy/jsu008

Kashikar-Zuck, S., Swain, N. F., Jones, B. A., & Graham, T. B. (2005). Efficacy of cognitive-behavioral intervention for juvenile primary fibromyalgia syndrome. *Journal of Rheumatology, 32*, 1594–1602.

Law, E. F., Fisher, E., Fales, J., Noel, M., & Eccleston, C. (2014). Systematic review and meta-analysis of parent and family-based interventions for children and adolescents with chronic medical conditions. *Journal of Pediatric Psychology, 39*, 866–886. http://dx.doi.org/10.1093/jpepsy/jsu032

Levy, R., Langer, S., Walker, L., Romano, J., Christie, D., Youssef, N., . . . Whitehead, W. (2010). Cognitive-behavioral therapy for children with functional abdominal pain and their parents decreases pain and other symptoms. *American Journal of Gastroenterology, 105,* 946–956. http://dx.doi.org/10.1038/ajg.2010.106

Palermo, T., Law, E., Fales, J., Bromberg, M., Jessen-Fiddick, T., & Tai, G. (2016). Internet-delivered cognitive-behavioral treatment for adolescents with chronic pain and their parents: A randomized controlled multicenter trial. *Pain, 157,* 174–185. http://dx.doi.org/10.1097/j.pain.0000000000000348

Powers, S. W., Kashikar-Zuck, S. M., Allen, J. R., LeCates, S. L., Slater, S. K., Zafar, M., . . . Hershey, A. D. (2013). Cognitive behavioral therapy plus amitriptyline for chronic migraine in children and adolescents: A randomized clinical trial. *JAMA, 310,* 2622–2630. http://dx.doi.org/10.1001/jama.2013.282533

Van Der Veek, S. M. C., Derkx, B. H., Benninga, M. A., Boer, F., & de Haan, E. (2013). Cognitive behavior therapy for pediatric functional abdominal pain: A randomized controlled trial. *Pediatrics, 132,* e1163–e1172. http://dx.doi.org/10.1542/peds.2013-0242

FIBROMYALGIA

Alba, M., Luciano, J. V., Andrés, E., Serrano-Blanco, A., Rodero, B., del Hoyo, Y. L., . . . García-Compayo, J. (2011). Effectiveness of cognitive behaviour therapy for treatment of catastrophisation in patients with fibromyalgia: A randomized controlled trial. *Arthritis Research & Therapy,13,* R173. http://dx.doi.org/10.1186/ar3496

Ang, D., Jensen, M., Steiner, J., Hilligoss, J., Gracely, R., & Saha, C. (2013). Combining cognitive-behavioral therapy and milnacipran for fibromyalgia: A feasibility randomized-controlled trial. *Clinical Journal of Pain, 29,* 747–754. http://dx.doi.org/10.1097/AJP.0b013e31827a784e

Bennett, R., & Nelson, D. (2006). Cognitive behavioral therapy for fibromyalgia. *Nature Clinical Practice Rheumatology, 2,* 416–424. http://dx.doi.org/10.1038/ncprheum0245

Bernardy, K., Klose, P., Busch, A. J., Choy, E. H. S., & Häuser, W. (2013). Cognitive behavioural therapies for fibromyalgia. *Cochrane Database of Systematic Reviews, 9,* CD009796. http://dx.doi.org/10.1002/14651858.CD009796.pub2

Fitzcharles, M.-A., Ste-Marie, P. A., Goldenberg, D. L., Pereira, J. X., Abbey, S., Choinière, M., . . . the National Fibromyalgia Guideline Advisory Panel. (2013). 2012 Canadian guidelines for the diagnosis and management of fibromyalgia syndrome: Executive summary. *Pain Research and Management, 18,* 119–126. http://dx.doi.org/10.1155/2013/918216

Luciano, J. V., D'Amico, F., Cerdà-Lafont, M., Peñarrubia-María, M. T., Knapp, M., Cuesta-Vargas, A. I., . . . García-Campayo, J. (2014). Cost-utility of cognitive behavioral therapy versus U.S. Food and Drug Administration recommended drugs and usual care in the treatment of patients with fibromyalgia: An economic evaluation alongside a 6-month randomized controlled trial. *Arthritis Research and Therapy, 16,* 451. http://dx.doi.org/10.1186/s13075-014-0451-y

Nuesch, E., Häuser, W., Bernardy, K., Barth, J., & Jüni, P. (2013). Comparative efficacy of pharmacological and non-pharmacological intervention in fibromyalgia syndrome: Network meta-analysis. *Annals of the Rheumatic Diseases, 72*, 955–962. http://dx.doi.org/10.1136/annrheumdis-2011-201249

HEADACHE

Andrasik, F. (2007). What does the evidence show? Efficacy of behavioural treatments for recurrent headaches in adults. *Neurological Sciences, 28*, S70–S77.

Harris, P., Loveman, E., Clegg, A. Easton, S., & Berry, N. (2015). Systematic review of cognitive behavioural therapy for the management of headaches and migraines in adults. *British Journal of Pain, 9*, 213–224. http://dx.doi.org/10.1177/2049463715578291

Holroyd, K. A., Penzien, D. B., Rains, J. C., Lipchik. G. L., & Buse, D. C. (2008). Behavioral management of headache. In S. D. Silberstein, R. B. Lipton, & D. W. Dodick (Eds.), *Wolff's headache: And other head pain* (8th ed., pp. 721–746). New York, NY: Oxford University Press.

Penzien, D. B., Irby, M. B., Smitherman, T. A., Rains, J. C., & Houle, T. T. (2015). Well-established and empirically supported behavioral treatments for migraine. *Current Pain and Headache Reports, 19*, 34. http://dx.doi.org/10.1007/s11916-015-0500-5

GASTROINTESTINAL DISORDERS/IRRITABLE BOWEL SYNDROME

Craske, M. G., Wolitzky-Taylor, K. B., Labus, J., Wu, S., Frese, M., Mayer, E. A., & Naliboff, B. D. (2011). A cognitive-behavioral treatment for irritable bowel syndrome using interoceptive exposure to visceral sensations. *Behaviour Research and Therapy, 49*, 413–421. http://dx.doi.org/10.1016/j.brat.2011.04.001

Labus, J., Gupta, A., Gill, H. K., Posserud, I., Mayer, M., Raeen, H., . . . Mayer, E. A. (2013). Randomised clinical trial: Symptoms of the irritable bowel syndrome are improved by a psycho-education group intervention. *Alimentary Pharmacology and Therapeutics, 37*, 304–315. http://dx.doi.org/10.1111/apt.12171

Lackner, J. M., Jaccard, J., Krasner, S. S., Katz, L. A., Gudleski, G. D., & Holroyd, K. (2008). Self-administered cognitive behavior therapy for moderate to severe irritable bowel syndrome: Clinical efficacy, tolerability, feasibility. *Clinical Gastroenterology and Hepatology, 6*, 899–906. http://dx.doi.org/10.1016/j.cgh.2008.03.004

Laird, K. T., Tanner-Smith, E. E., Russell, A. C., Hollon, S. D., & Walker, L. S. (2016). Short-term and long-term efficacy of psychological therapies for irritable bowel syndrome: A systematic review and meta-analysis. *Clinical Gastroenterology and Hepatology, 14*, 937–947. http://dx.doi.org/10.1016/j.cgh.2015.11.020

Li, L., Xiong, L., Zhang, S., Yu, Q., & Chen, M. (2014). Cognitive-behavioral therapy for irritable bowel syndrome: A meta-analysis. *Journal of Psychosomatic Research, 77*, 1–12. http://dx.doi.org/10.1016/j.jpsychores.2014.03.006

Van Dulmen, A. M., Fennis, J. F., & Bleijenberg, G. (1996). Cognitive-behavioral group therapy for irritable bowel syndrome: Effects and long-term follow-up. *Psychosomatic Medicine, 58*, 508–514. http://dx.doi.org/10.1097/00006842-199609000-00013

MUSCULOSKELETAL PAIN (MIXED)

Du, S., Yuan, C., Xiao, X., Chu, J., Qiu, Y., & Qian, H. (2011). Self-management programs for chronic musculoskeletal pain conditions: A systematic review and meta-analysis. *Patient Education and Counseling, 85*, e299–e310. http://dx.doi.org/10.1016/j.pec.2011.02.021

CHRONIC PAIN AND COMORBID MEDICAL CONDITIONS

Morasco, B. J., Greaves, D. W., Lovejoy, T. I., Turk, D. C., Dobscha, S. K., & Hauser, P. (2016). Development and preliminary evaluation of an integrated cognitive-behavior treatment for chronic pain in patients and substance use disorder in patients with hepatitis C virus. *Pain Medicine, 17*, 2280–2290. http://dx.doi.org/10.1093/pm/pnw076

Morasco, B. J., Gritzner, S., Lewis, L., Oldham, R., Turk, D. C., & Dobscha, S. K. (2011). Systematic review of prevalence, correlates, and treatment outcomes for chronic non-cancer pain in patients with comorbid substance use disorder. *Pain, 152*, 488–497. http://dx.doi.org/10.1016/j.pain.2010.10.009

Otis, J. D., Keane, T. M., Kerns, R. D., Monson, C., & Scioli, E. (2009). The development of an integrated treatment for veterans with comorbid chronic pain and posttraumatic stress disorder. *Pain Medicine, 10*, 1300–1311. http://dx.doi.org/10.1111/j.1526-4637.2009.00715.x

Substance Abuse and Mental Health Services Administration. (2011). Managing chronic pain in adults with or in recovery from substance use disorders [Treatment Improvement Protocol (TIP) Series 54:HHS Publication No. (SMA) 12-4671]. Rockville, MD: Author.

Thorn, B. E., Day, M. A., Burns, J., Kuhajda, M. C., Gaskins, S. W., Sweeney, K., McConley, R., Ward, L. C., & Cabbil, C. (2011). Randomized trial of group cognitive behavioral therapy compared with pain education control for low-literacy rural people with chronic pain. *Pain, 152*, 2710–2720. http://dx.doi.org/10.1016/j.pain.2011.07.007

NONCARDIAC CHEST PAIN

Keefe, F. J., Shelby, R. A., Somers, T. J., Varia, I., Blazing, M., Waters, S. J., . . . Bradley, L. (2011). Effects of coping skills training and sertraline in patients with non-cardiac chest pain: A randomized controlled study. *Pain, 152*, 730–741. http://dx.doi.org/10.1016/j.pain.2010.08.040

Van Peski-Oosterbaan, A. S., Spinhoven, P., Van der Does, A. J., Bruschke, A. V., & Rooijmans, H. G. M. (1999). Cognitive change following cognitive behavioural therapy for non-cardiac chest pain. *Psychotherapy and Psychosomatics, 68*, 214–220. http://dx.doi.org/10.1159/000012335

Van Peski-Oosterbaan, A. S., Spinhoven, P., van Rood, Y., van der Does, J. W., Bruschke, A. V., Rooijmans, H. G. (1999). Cognitive-behavioral therapy for noncardiac chest pain: A randomized trial. *American Journal of Medicine 106*, 424–429. http://dx.doi.org/10.1016/S0002-9343(99)00049-2

PAIN IN OLDER ADULTS

Barefoot, C., Hadjistavropoulos, T. D., Carleton, R. N., & Henry, J. (2012). A brief report on the evaluation of a pain self-management program for older adults. *Journal of Cognitive Psychotherapy, 26,* 157–168. http://dx.doi.org/10.1891/0889-8391.26.2.157

Green, S. M., Hadjistavropoulos, T., Hadjistavropoulos, H., Martin, R., & Sharpe, D. (2009). A controlled investigation of a cognitive behavioural pain management program for older adults. *Behavioural and Cognitive Psychotherapy, 37,* 221–226. http://dx.doi.org/10.1017/S1352465809005177

Hadjistavropoulos, T. (2012). Self-management of pain in older persons: Helping people help themselves. *Pain Medicine, 13*(Suppl.), S67–S71. http://dx.doi.org/10.1111/j.1526-4637.2011.01272.x

Hadjistavropoulos, T., & Hadjistavropoulos, H. D. (Eds.). (2008). *Pain management in older adults: A self-help guide.* Seattle, WA: IASP Press.

Keefe, F. J., Porter, L., Somers, T., Shelby, R., & Wren, A. V. (2013). Psychosocial interventions for managing pain in older adults: Outcomes and clinical implications. *British Journal of Anaesthesia, 111,* 89–94. http://dx.doi.org/10.1093/bja/aet129

Lunde, L.-H., Nordhus, I. H., & Pallesen, S. (2009). The effectiveness of cognitive and behavioural treatment of chronic pain in the elderly: A quantitative review. *Journal of Clinical Psychology in Medical Settings, 16,* 254–262. http://dx.doi.org/10.1007/s10880-009-9162-y

McGuire, B. E., Nicholas, M. K., Asghari, A., Wood, B. M., & Main, C. J. (2014). The effectiveness of psychological treatments for chronic pain in older adults: Cautious optimism and an agenda for research. *Current Opinion in Psychiatry, 27,* 380–384. http://dx.doi.org/10.1097/YCO.0000000000000090

Nicholas, M. K., Asghari, A., Blyth, F. M., Wood, B. M., Murray, R., McCabe, R., . . . Overton, S. (2013). Self-management intervention for chronic pain in older adults: A randomized controlled trial. *Pain, 154,* 824–835. http://dx.doi.org/10.1016/j.pain.2013.02.009

PELVIC PAIN

Bergeron, S., Khalifé, S., Dupuis, M.-J., & McDuff, P. (2016). A randomized clinical trial comparing group cognitive-behavioral therapy and a topical steroid for women with dyspareunia. *Journal of Consulting and Clinical Psychology, 84,* 259–268. http://dx.doi.org/10.1037/ccp0000072

Corsini-Munt, S., Bergeron, S., Rosen, N. O., Mayrand, M.-H., & Delisle, I. (2014). Feasibility and preliminary effectiveness of a novel cognitive–behavioral couple therapy for provoked vestibulodynia: A pilot study. *Journal of Sexual Medicine, 11,* 2515–2527. http://dx.doi.org/10.1111/jsm.12646

Goldfinger, C., Pukall, C. F., Thibault-Gagnon, S., McLean, L., & Chamberlain, S. (2016). Effectiveness of cognitive-behavioral therapy and physical therapy for provoked vestibulodynia: A randomized pilot study. *Journal of Sexual Medicine, 13,* 88–94. http://dx.doi.org/10.1016/j.jsxm.2015.12.003

Masheb, R. M., Kerns, R. D., Lozano, C., Minkin, M. J., & Richman, S. (2009). A randomized clinical trial for women with vulvodynia: Cognitive-behavioral therapy vs. supportive psychotherapy. *Pain, 141*, 31–49. http://dx.doi.org/10.1016/j.pain.2008.09.031

TEMPOROMANDIBULAR DISORDERS

Aggawal, V. R., Fu, Y., Main, C. J., & Wu, J. (2019). The effectiveness of self-management interventions in adults with chronic orofacial pain: A systematic review, meta-analysis, and meta-regression. *European Journal of Pain, 23*, 849–865.

Bogart, R. K., McDaniel, R. J., Dunn, W. J., Hunter, C., Peterson, A. L., & Wright, E. F. (2007). Efficacy of group cognitive behavior therapy for the management of masticatory myofascial pain. *Military Medicine, 172*, 169–174. http://dx.doi.org/10.7205/milmed.172.2.169

Mishra, K. D., Gatchel, R. J., & Gardea, M. A. (2000). The relative efficacy of three cognitive-behavioral treatment approaches to temporomandibular disorders. *Journal of Behavioral Medicine, 23*, 293–309. http://dx.doi.org/10.1023/a:1005562126071

Orlando, B., Manfredini, D., Salvetti, G., & Bosco, M. (2007). Evaluation of the effectiveness of biobehavioral therapy in the treatment of temporomandibular disorders: A literature review. *Behavioral Medicine, 33*, 101–118. http://dx.doi.org/10.3200/BMED.33.3.101-118

Shedden Mora, M. C., Weber, D., Neff, A., & Rief, W. (2013). Biofeedback-based cognitive-behavioral treatment compared with occlusal splint for temporomandibular disorder: A randomized controlled trial. *Clinical Journal of Pain, 29*, 1057–1065. http://dx.doi.org/10.1097/AJP.0b013e3182850559

Turner, J. A., Mancl, L., & Aaron, L. A. (2006). Short- and long-term efficacy of brief cognitive-behavioral therapy for patients with chronic temporomandibular disorder: A randomized, controlled trial. *Pain, 121*, 181–194. http://dx.doi.org/10.1016/j.pain.2005.11.017

WHIPLASH INJURY (NECK AND SHOULDER PAIN) FOLLOWING MOTOR VEHICLE ACCIDENTS

Dunne, R., Kenardy, J., & Sterling, M. (2012). A randomized controlled trial of cognitive-behavioral therapy for the treatment of PTSD in the context of chronic whiplash. *Clinical Journal of Pain, 28*, 755–765. http://dx.doi.org/10.1097/AJP.0b013e318243e16b

Linton, S. J. (2016). Improving psychologically oriented treatments for WAD. In H. Kasch, D. C. Turk, & T. S. Jensen (Eds.). *Whiplash injury: Perspectives on the development of chronic pain* (pp. 189–208). Washington, DC: IASP press.

REFERENCES

Abdel Shaheed, C., Maher, G., Williams, K., & McLachlan, A. J. (2017). Efficacy and tolerability of muscle relaxants for low back pain: Systemic review and meta-analysis. *European Journal of Pain, 21*, 228–237.

Adachi, T., Fujino, H., Nkae, A., Mashimo, T., & Sasaki, S. (2014). A meta-analysis of hypnosis for chronic pain problems: A comparison between hypnosis, standard care, and other psychological interventions. *International Journal of Clinical and Experimental Hypnosis, 62*, 1–28.

Angarita, G. A., Emadi, N., Hodges, S., & Morgan, P. T. (2016). Sleep abnormalities associated with alcohol, cannabis, cocaine, and opiate use: A comprehensive review. *Addiction Science & Clinical Practice, 11*, 9. Advance online publication. http://dx.doi.org/10.1186/s13722-016-0056-7

Ashburn, M. A., & Fleisher, L. A. (2018, December 18). Increasing evidence for the limited role of opioids to treat chronic noncancer pain. *JAMA, 320*(23), 2427–2428. http://dx.doi.org/10.1001/jama.2018.19327

Babalonis, S., Lofwall, M. R., Nuzzo, P., Siegel, A. J., & Walsh, S. L. (2013). Abuse liability and reinforcing efficacy of oral tramadol in humans. *Drug and Alcohol Dependence, 129*, 116–124.

Bannuru, R. R., Schmid, C. H., Kent, D. M., Vaysbrot, E. E., Wong, J. B., & McAlindon, T. E. (2015). Comparative effectiveness of pharmacologic interventions for knee osteoarthritis. A systematic review and network meta-analysis. *Annals of Internal Medicine, 162*, 46–54. http://dx.doi.org/10.7326/M14-1231

Bhala, N., Emberson, J., Merhi, A., Abramson, S., Arber, S., Baron, J. A., . . . Baigent, C. (2013). Vascular and upper gastrointestinal effects of non-steroidal anti-inflammatory drugs: Meta-analyses of individual participant data from randomised trials. *The Lancet, 382*(9894), 769–779. http://dx.doi.org/10.1016/S0140-6736(13)60900-9

Brosseau, L., Yonge, K. A., Welch, V., Marchand, S., Judd, M., Wells, G. A., & Tugwell, P. (2003). Thermotherapy for treatment of osteoarthritis. *Cochrane Database of Systematic Reviews*, CD004522. Advance online publication. http://dx.doi.org/10.1002/14651858.CD004522

Brunton, S., Wang, F., Edwards, S. B., Crucitti, A. S., Ossanna, M. J., Walker, D. J., & Robinson, M. J. (2010). Profiles of adverse events with duloxetine treatment: A pooled analysis of placebo-controlled studies. *Drug Safety, 33*, 393–407. http://dx.doi.org/10.2165/11319200-000000000-00000

Buchmuller, A., Navez, M., Milletre-Bernardin, M., Pouplin, S., Presles, E., Lantéri-Minet, M., . . . Camdessanché, J. P. (2012). Value of TENS for relief of chronic low back pain with or without radicular pain. *European Journal of Pain, 16*, 656–665. http://dx.doi.org/10.1002/j.1532-2149.2011.00061.x

Busch, A. J., Barber, K. A., Overend, T. J., Peloso, P. M., & Schachter, C. L. (2007). Exercise for treating fibromyalgia syndrome. *Cochrane Database of Systematic Reviews, 4*, CD003786.

Buse, J. W., Wang, L., Kamaleldin, M., Craigie, S., Riva, J. J., Montoya, L., . . . Guyatt, G. H. (2018, December 18). Opioids for chronic noncancer pain: A systematic review and meta-analysis. *JAMA, 320*, 2448–2460. http://dx.doi.org/10.1001/jama.2018.18472

Bush, D. M. (2015). Emergency department visits for adverse reactions involving the pain medication tramadol. *The CBHSQ Report.* Retrieved from https://www.ncbi.nlm.nih.gov/books/NBK343538/

Cheatle, M. D., & Shmuts, R. (2015). The risk and benefit of benzodiazepine use in patients with chronic pain. *Pain Medicine, 16*, 219–221.

Chou, R., McDonagh, M. S., Nakamoto, E., & Griffin, J. (2011). *Analgesics for osteoarthritis: An update of the 2006 comparative effectiveness review.* Rockville, MD: Agency for Healthcare Research and Quality.

Chou, R., Turner, J. A., Devine, E. B., Hansen, R. N., Sullivan, S. D., Blazina, I., . . . Deyo, R. A. (2015). The effectiveness and risks of long-term opioid therapy for chronic pain: A systematic review for a National Institutes of Health Pathways to Prevention Workshop. *Annals of Internal Medicine, 162*, 267–286. http://dx.doi.org/10.7326/M14-2559

Cramer, H., Lauche, R., Haller, H., & Dubos, G. (2013). A systematic review and meta-analysis of yoga for low back pain. *Clinical Journal of Pain, 29*, 450–460.

Derry, S., Conaghan, P., Da Silva, J. A. P., Wiffen, P. J., & Moore, R. A. (2016). Topical NSAIDs for chronic musculoskeletal pain in adults. *Cochrane Database of Systematic Review, 4*, CD007400. http://dx.doi.org/10.1002/14651858.CD007400.pub3

Derry, S., Wiffen, P., Moore, R., & Guinlan, J. (2014). Topical lidocaine for neuropathic pain in adults. *Cochrane Database of Systematic Reviews, 7*, 1–50.

DeSantana, J. M., Walsh, D. M., Vance, C., Rakel, B. A., & Saluka, K. A. (2008). Effectiveness of transcutaneous electrical nerve stimulation for treatment of hyperalgesia and pain. *Current Rheumatology Reports, 10*, 492–499.

Dowell, D., Haegerich, T. M., & Chou, R. (2016, April 19). CDC guideline for prescribing opioids for chronic pain—United States, 2016. *JAMA, 315*, 1624–1645. http://dx.doi.org/10.1001/jama.2016.1464

Ebadi, S., Henschke, N., Nakhostin Ansari, N., Fall, E., & van Tulder, M. W. (2014). Therapeutic ultrasound for chronic low-back pain. *Cochrane Database of Systematic Reviews*, CD009169.

Ehde, D. M., Dillworth, T. M., & Turner, J. A. (2014). Cognitive-behavioral therapy for individuals with chronic pain: Efficacy, innovations and directions for research. *American Psychologist, 69*, 153–166. http://dx.doi.org/10.1037/a0035747

Epstein, N. E. (2013). The risks of epidural and transforaminal steroid injections in the spine: Commentary and a comprehensive review of the literature. *Surgical Neurology International, 4*, S74–S93. http://dx.doi.org/10.4103/2F2152-7806.109446

Flor, H., & Turk, D. C. (2011). *Chronic pain: An integrated biobehavioral perspective.* Seattle, WA: IASP Press.

Franklin, G., Haug, J., Heyer, N. J., McKeefrey, S. P., & Picciano, J. F. (1994). Outcome of lumbar fusion in Washington State Workers' Compensation. *Spine, 19,* 1897–1904.

French, S. D., Cameron, M., Walker, F., Reggars, J. W., & Esterman, A. J. (2006). Superficial heat or cold for low back pain. *Cochrane Database of Systematic Reviews,* CD004750. http://dx.doi.org/10.1002/14651858.CD004750.pub2

Furlan, A. D., Imamura, M., Dryden, T., & Irvin, E. (2008). Massage for low-back pain. *Cochrane Database of Systematic Review,* CD0011929.

Furlan, A. D., Sandoval, J. A., Mailis-Gagnon, A., & Tunks, E. (2006). Opioids for chronic noncancer pain: A meta-analysis of effectiveness and side effects. *Canadian Medical Association Journal, 174,* 1589–1594.

Galer, B., Rowbotham, M., Perander, J., & Friedman, E. (1999). Topical lidocaine patch relieves postherpetic neuralgia more effectively than a vehicle topical patch: Results of an enriched enrollment study. *Pain, 80,* 533–538. http://dx.doi.org/10.1016/S0304-3959(98)00244-9

Gauntlett-Gilbert, J., Gavriloff, D., & Brook, P. (2016). Benzodiazepines may be worse than opioids: Negative medication effects in severe chronic pain. *Clinical Journal of Pain, 32,* 285–289.

Hall, A. M., Maher, C. G., Lam, O., Ferreira, M., & Latimer, J. (2011). Tai chi exercise for treatment of pain and disability in people with persistent low back pain: A randomized controlled trial. *Arthritis Care and Research, 63,* 1576–1583.

Hayden, J. A., van Tulder, M. W., Malmivara, A., & Koes, B. W. (2005). Exercise therapy for treatment of non-specific low back pain. *Cochrane Database of Systematic Reviews, 3,* CD000355. http://dx.doi.org/10.1002/14651858.CD000335.pub2

Herndon, C. M., Hutchinson, R. W., Berdine, H. J., Stacey, Z. A., Chen, J. T., Farnsworth, D. D., . . . Fermo, J. D. (2008). Management of chronic nonmalignant pain with nonsteroidal anti-inflammatory drugs: Joint opinion statement of the Ambulatory Care, Cardiology, and Pain and Palliative Care Practice and Research Networks of the American College of Clinical Pharmacy. *Pharmacotherapy, 28,* 788–805. http://dx.doi.org/10.1592/phco.28.6.788

Hilton, L., Hempel, S., Ewing, B. A., Apaydin, E., Xenakis, L., Newberry, S., . . . Maglione, M. A. (2017). Mindfulness meditation for chronic pain: Systematic review and meta-analysis. *Annals of Behavioral Medicine, 51,* 199–213. http://dx.doi.org/10.1007/s12160-016-9844-2

Hughes, L. S., Clark, J., Colclough, J. A., Dale, E., & McMillan, D. (2017). Acceptance and commitment therapy (ACT) for chronic pain: A systematic review and meta-analysis. *Clinical Journal of Pain, 33,* 552–568.

Jensen, M. P., & Patterson, D. R. (2014). Hypnotic approaches for chronic pain management: Clinical implications of research findings. *American Psychologist, 69,* 167–177. http://dx.doi.org/10.1037/a0035644

Jones, V. M., Moore, K. A., & Peterson, D. M. (2011). Capsaicin 8% topical patch (Qutenza)—a review of the evidence. *Journal of Pain and Palliative Care Pharmacotherapy, 25,* 32–41. http://dx.doi.org/10.3109/15360288.2010.547561

Kamper, S. J., Apeldoorn, A. T., Chiarotto, A., Smeets, R. J. E. M., Ostelo, R. W. J. G., Guzman, J., & van Tulder, M. W. (2014). Multidisciplinary biopsychosocial rehabilitation for chronic low back pain. *Cochrane Database of Systematic Reviews,* CD000963. Advance online publication. http://dx.doi.org/10.1002/14651858.CD000963.pub3

Kerns, R. D., Turk, D. C., & Rudy, T. E. (1985). The West Haven-Yale Multidimensional Pain Inventory (WHYMPI). *Pain, 23,* 345–356.

Kortebein, P., Ferrando, A., Lombeida, J., Wolfe, R., & Evans, W. J. (2007, April 25). Effect of 10 days of bed rest on skeletal muscle in healthy older adults. *JAMA, 297,* 1772–1774. http://dx.doi.org/10.1001/jama.297.16.1772-b

Kumar, K., Hunter, G., & Demeria, D. (2006). Spinal cord stimulation in treatment of chronic benign pain: Challenges in treatment planning and present status, a 22-year experience. *Neurosurgery, 58,* 481–496. http://dx.doi.org/10.1227/01.NEU.0000192162.99567.96

Lam, M., Galvin, R., & Curry, P. (2013). Effectiveness of acupuncture for non-specific chronic low back pain: A systematic review and meta-analysis. *Spine, 38,* 2124–2138. http://dx.doi.org/10.1097/01.brs.0000435025.65564.b7

Luijsterburg, P. A. J., Ostelo, R. W., Verhagen, A., & Van Os, T. A. G. (2007). Effectiveness of conservative treatments for the lumbosacral radicular syndrome: A systematic review. *European Spine Journal, 16,* 881–899. http://dx.doi.org/10.1007/s00586-007-0367-1

Marsico, F., Paolillo, S., & Filardi, P. P. (2017). NSAIDs and cardiovascular risk. *Journal of Cardiovascular Medicine, 18,* e40–e43. http://dx.doi.org/10.2459/JCM.0000000000000443

McPherson, M. L., & Cimino, N. M. (2013). Topical NSAID formulations. *Pain Medicine, 14,* S35–S39. http://dx.doi.org/10.1111/pme.12288

Merrill, D. G. (2003). Hoffman's glasses: Evidence-based medicine and the search for quality in the literature of interventional pain medicine. *Regional Anesthesia and Pain Medicine, 28,* 547–560.

Moore, R. A., Derry, S., Aldington, D., Cole, P., & Wiffen, P. J. (2015). Amitriptyline for neuropathic pain in adults. *Cochrane Database of Systematic Reviews, 7,* DC008242.

Nestoriuc, Y., Martin, A. Rief, W., & Andrasik, F. (2008). Biofeedback treatment for headache disorders: A comprehensive efficacy review. *Applied Psychophysiology and Biofeedback, 33,* 125–140. http://dx.doi.org/10.1007/s10484-008-9060-3

North American Spine Society. (2007). *Diagnosis and treatment of degenerative lumbar spinal stenosis.* Retrieved from https://www.spine.org/Portals/0/assets/downloads/ResearchClinicalCare/Guidelines/LumbarStenosis.pdf

Nugent, S. M., Morasco, B. J., O'Neil, M. E., Freeman, M., Low, A., Kondo, K., . . . Kansagara, D. (2017). The effects of cannabis among adults with chronic pain and an overview of general harms: A systematic review. *Annals of Internal Medicine, 167,* 319–331. http://dx.doi.org/10.7326/M17-0155

Penzien, D., Irby, M., Smitherman, T., Rains, J. C., & Houle, T. T. (2015). Well-established and empirically supported behavioral treatments for migraine. *Current Pain and Headache Reports, 19,* 34. http://dx.doi.org/10.1007/s11916-015-0500-5

Pinto, R. Z., Maher, C. G., Ferreira, M. L., Hancock, M., Oliveira, V. C., McLachlan, A. J., . . . Ferreira, P. H. (2012). Epidural corticosteroid injections in the management of sciatica: A systematic review and meta-analysis. *Annals of Internal Medicine, 157,* 865–877. http://dx.doi.org/10.7326/0003-4819-157-12-201212180-00564

Reiner, K., Tibi, L., & Lipsitz, J. D. (2013). Do mindfulness-based interventions reduce pain intensity? A critical review of the literature. *Pain Medicine, 14,* 230–242. http://dx.doi.org/10.1111/pme.12006

Richards, B., Whittle, S., & Buchbinder, R. (2011). Antidepressants for pain management in rheumatoid arthritis. *Cochrane Data Base of Systematic Reviews, 11,* CD008920.

Rosenow, J. M., Stanton-Hicks, M., Rezai, A. R., & Henderson, J. M. (2006). Failure modes of spinal cord stimulation hardware. *Journal of Neurosurgery Spine, 5,* 183–190. http://dx.doi.org/10.3171/spi.2006.5.3.183

Ross, A., & Thomas, S. (2010). The health benefits of yoga and exercise: A review of comparison studies. *Journal of Alternative and Complementary Medicine, 16,* 3–12. http://dx.doi.org/10.1089/acm.2009.0044

Rubinstein, S. M., de Zoetz, A., Van Middelkoop, M., Assendelft, W. J. J., de Boer, M. R., & van Tulder, M. W. (2019, March 13). Benefits and harms of spinal manipulative therapy for the treatment of chronic low back pain: Systematic review and meta-analysis of randomized controlled trials. *BMJ, 364,* 1689. http://dx.doi.org/10.1136/bmj.l689

Saarto, T., & Wiffen, P. (2007). Antidepressants for neuropathic pain. *Cochrane Database of Systematic Reviews, 4,* CD005454.

Saragiotto, B. T., Machado, G. C., Ferreira, M. L., Pinheiro, M. B., Abdel Shaheed, C., & Maher, C. G. (2016). Paracetamol for low back pain. *Cochrane Database of Systematic Reviews, 6,* CD012239. http://dx.doi.org/10.1002/14651858.CD012230

Scott, N. A., Guo, B., Barton, P. M., & Gerwin, R. D. (2009). Trigger point injections for chronic non-malignant musculoskeletal pain: A systematic review. *Pain Medicine, 10,* 54–69. http://dx.doi.org/10.1111/j.1526-4637.2008.00526.x

Smith, R. B., Havens, J. R., & Walsh, S. L. (2016). Gabapentin misuse, abuse and diversion: A systematic review. *Addiction, 111,* 1160–1174. http://dx.doi.org/10.1111/add.13324

Stockings, E., Campbell, G., Hall, W. D., & Nielsen, S. (2018). Cannabis and cannabinoids for the treatment of people with chronic noncancer pain conditions: Systematic review and meta-analysis of controlled and observational studies. *Pain, 159,* 1932–1954. http://dx.doi.org/10.1097/j.pain.0000000000001293

Turk, D. C. (2018). A cognitive-behavioral perspective on the treatment of individuals experiencing chronic pain. In D. C. Turk & R. J. Gatchel (Eds.), *Psychological approaches to pain management: A practitioner's handbook* (3rd ed., pp. 115–137). New York, NY: Guilford Press.

Turk, D. C., Wilson, H. D., & Cahana, A. (2011). Treatment of chronic noncancer pain. *The Lancet, 377,* 2226–2235. http://dx.doi.org/10.1016/S0140-6736(11)60402-9

Turner, J. A., Hollingworth, W., Comstock, B., & Deyo, R. (2010). Spinal cord stimulation for failed back surgery syndrome: Outcomes in a workers' compensation setting. *Pain, 148,* 14–25. http://dx.doi.org/10.1016/j.pain.2009.08.014

Urquhart, D. M., Hoving, J. L., Assendefft, W. W., Roland, M., & van Tulder, M. W. (2008). Antidepressants for non-specific low back pain. *Cochrane Database of Systematic Reviews, 1,* CD001703. http://dx.doi.org/10.1002/14651858.CD001703.pub3

Veehof, M. H., Trompetter, H. R., Bohlmeijer, E. T., & Schreurs, K. M. G. (2016). Acceptance-and mindfulness-based interventions for the treatment of chronic pain: A meta-analytic review. *Cognitive Behaviour Therapy, 45,* 5–31. http://dx.doi.org/10.1080/16506073.2015.1098724

Wang, Z. Y., Shi, S. Y., Li, S. J., Chen, F., Chen, H., Lin, H. Z., & Lin, J. M. (2015). Efficacy and safety of duloxetine on osteoarthritis knee pain: A meta-analysis of randomized controlled trials. *Pain Medicine, 16,* 1373–1385. http://dx.doi.org/10.1111/pme.12800

Wasan, A. D., Jamison, R. N., Pham, L., Tipirneni, N., Nedeljkovic, S. S., & Katz, J. N. (2009). Psychopathology predicts the outcome of medial branch blocks with corticosteroid for chronic axial low back or cervical pain: A prospective cohort study. *BMC Musculoskeletal Disorders, 10,* 22. http://dx.doi.org/10.1186/1471-2474-10-22

Wells, C., Kolt, G. S., Marshall, P., Hill, B., & Bialocerkowski, A. (2014). The effectiveness of Pilates exercise in people with chronic low back pain: A systematic review. *PLoS One,* e100402. http://dx.doi.org/10.1371/journal.pone.0100402

Wiffen, P. J., Derry, S., Moore, R. A., Aldington, D., Cole, P., Rice, A. S. C., . . . Kalso, E. A. (2013). Antiepileptic drugs for neuropathic pain and fibromyalgia—an overview of Cochrane reviews. *Cochrane Database of Systematic Reviews, 11,* CD010567. http://dx.doi.org/10.1002/14651858.CD010567.pub2

Williams, A. C., Eccleston, C., & Morley, S. (2012). Psychological therapies for the management of chronic pain (excluding headache) in adults. *Cochrane Database of*

Systemic Reviews, 11, CD007407. http://dx.doi.org/10.1002/14651858.CD007407.
pub3

Zhang, S.-S., Wu, Z., Zhang, L.-C., Zhang, Z., Chen, R.-P., Huang, Y.-H., & Chen, H.
(2015). Efficacy and safety of pregabalin for painful diabetic peripheral neuropathy: A meta-analysis. *Acta Anaesthesiologica Scandinavica, 59*(2), 147–159. http://
dx.doi.org/10.1111/aas.12420

Zhao, P., Yoo, I., Lancey, R., & Varghese, E. (2019). Mobile applications for pain
management: An app analysis for clinical usage. *BMC Medical Informatics and
Decision Making, 19,* 106. http://dx.doi.org/10.1186/s12911-019-0827-7

INDEX

A

ABCD coping model, 138–141
Acceptance, 147–149, 177
Acceptance and commitment therapy (ACT), 190
Acetaminophen, 184–185
ACPA (American Chronic Pain Association), 85, 201
ACT (acceptance and commitment therapy), 190
Active coping strategies, 28
Acupuncture, 184
Acute injuries
  expected healing for, 13
  and physical movement, 20
  rest subsequent to, 28
Aerobic exercise, 192
Aggression, 98
Airing Pain podcast, 202
Alcohol use
  and denial of limitations, 147
  and personal responsibility, 164
  and reinforcement, 119
  relaxation with, 56–57
  and sleep quality, 79, 80
Allen, James, 164
Allergies, 56
All-or-nothing approaches, 42
American Chronic Pain Association (ACPA), 85, 201
American College of Sports Medicine, 194
American Geriatrics Society, 202
American Migraine Association, 204

Amitryptiline, 186
Amputation, 15
Analgesic medication, 20–21, 184–185.
  See also Opioids
Anesthesia, 17
Anger
  and behavioral change, 118
  behavior related to, 134
  and responses from others, 6
  and self-confidence, 148
Annoyance, 118
Antianxiety medications, 56–57
Antibiotic drugs, 7
Anticonvulsants, 185
Antidepressant drugs, 57, 186
Anxiety
  and communication, 100
  medications for, 192
  in past and present, 162
  and threat, 16
Apps (smartphone applications), 37, 81, 201
Archaeology, 166
Art, 173
Arthritis, 7, 13, 203
Arthritis Foundation, 203
Assertion, 97, 98
Ativan (lorazepam), 192
Attention, 112–118, 120, 173
Attention diversion, 60–61
Atwood, Margaret, 73
Audio relaxation tools, 57, 58
Automatic behaviors, 110

Autonomy, 156
Avoidance behavior, 122
Avoidance learning, 113

B

Back pain
  biofeedback for treatment of, 187
  expected healing for, 13
  and fatigue, 76
  online resources for, 203
  and physical movement, 35
  and Pilates, 192
  research on management of, 7
  steroid treatment for, 189
  unidentifiable causes of, 14
Balance
  and fatigue, 73
  and physical movement, 30–31
  and self-confidence, 154
"Balanced growth," 81–82
Baseline (physical movement), 36–37, 43
Baths, 80
Bedtime rituals, 80
Behavioral change, 109–125
  and attention, 112–118, 120
  for changing mood, 133–134
  and laws of learning, 109, 114–115
  preparation for, 122–123
  reinforcement for, 110–112, 114, 118–122
Behavioral communication, 99–101
Biofeedback, 187
Biomedical approaches, 20
Black-and-white thinking, 130
Blaming thoughts, 129
Board games, 173
Bodily experiences, 53
Body language, 93, 97
Boredom, 172
Bowel problems, 55
Breathing
  controlled, 69–70
  in Pilates, 192
  practicing of, 179
  and relaxation techniques, 51, 58–60
Bruner, Jerome, 109

C

Caffeine, 80
Cancer
  and opioids, 3
  pain associated with, 13, 14
Candles, 178
Cannabidiol (CBD), 187–188
Cannabis, 187–188
Capsaicin (Quienza), 195
Car repair, 173

Catastrophizing, 130
CAT (computed axial tomography) scans, 14
CBD (cannabidiol), 187–188
CBT (cognitive behavior therapy), 188, 190
Cell phones, 50
Change, 74
Chemotherapy, 14
Chiropractors, 193
Chronic fatigue, 55
Chronic pain. *See also* Pain
  nature of, 13–16
  prevalence of, 13
  and rest, 28
Chronic regional pain syndrome, 193
Clonazepam (Klonopin), 192
Club memberships, 173
CNET (website), 201
Cochrane Database of Systematic Review, 183
Cognitive behavior therapy (CBT), 188, 190
Cognitive functioning, 54–55
Cold therapy, 195
Comfort foods, 77–78
Communication, 89–107
  behavioral, 99–101
  common problems with, 93–96
  home activities for, 105
  importance of, 89–92, 179
  and pain assessment, 106–107
  partner intimacy as, 101–103
  questions to consider with, 104
  and sharing with others, 92–93
  strategies for improvement of, 96–98
Community resources, 85, 173
Compromise, 98
Computerized axial tomography (CAT) scans, 14
Concentration difficulties, 54–55
Conflict, 127–128
Consumer Reports, 201
Control, 85, 151–152
Control fallacies, 130
Cooking, 84
Corticosteroids, 196
Crafts, 84, 173
Creative outlets, 84
Crohn's disease, 205
Curie, Marie, 145
Cyclobenzaprine (Flexeril), 192
Cymbalta (duloxetine), 186

D

Data collection, 28
Dental care, 54
Depression
  and antidepressants, 186
  and behavioral change, 118

as common experience with chronic
    pain, 16
and others' responses to pain, 6
and self-confidence, 148
and sleep quality, 79
Desirability, 119
Despondency, 148
Diaphragmatic breathing, 58–59
Diathermy, 192
Diazepam (Valium), 192
Diclofenac, 195
Dietary changes, 123, 161
Dieting, 34
Digestive problems, 55–56
DIPEx International, 202
Disability payments, 6, 14
Diversion activities, 60–61, 84, 172
Drama activities, 173
Drawing, 84, 173
Drug use, 56–57
Duloxetine (Cymbalta), 186

E

Effexor (venlafaxine), 186
Electrical stimulation, 193, 195–196
Embarrassment, 118
Emotional reasoning, 130
Emotional tiredness, 74–75
Emotional vulnerability, 53–54
Emotion management, 28
Emotions
    and behavioral change, 118
    and eating, 78
    stressful. *See* Stressful thoughts and
        feelings
Endometriosis, 203, 205
Endometriosis UK, 203
Endorphins, 77
Endurance, 76
Energy balance, 50–51
Energy conservation, 52
Entitlement fallacy, 130–131
Epidural block, 191
Epidural steroids injections (ESIs), 189
Erving, Maria, 49
Exercise. *See* Physical movement
Exercise physiologists, 192
Exertion, 33, 40
Expectations, 82–84

F

Facial neuropathy, 193
Facial pain, 187
Failed back surgery syndrome, 193
Family members
    negative effects of, 6, 41–42
    sharing with, 91–92. *See also*
        Communication

Fatigue, 73–88
    behavior related to, 134
    and emotional tiredness, 74–75
    home activities for management of,
        87–88
    and improvement of sleep, 79–81
    and nutritional tiredness, 77–79
    pacing for management of, 81–82
    and physical tiredness, 75–77
    questions to consider with, 86
    and relaxation techniques, 55
    and self-expectations, 82–84
    strategies for management of, 84–85
Fear
    and behavioral change, 118
    behavior related to, 134
    and relaxation techniques, 54
Fibromyalgia
    biofeedback for treatment of, 187
    exercise for, 192
    online resources for, 203
    prevalence of pain with, 13
    research on management of, 7
    and unidentifiable causes of pain, 14
Fight-or-flight mode, 129
Filtering (thinking error), 130
Financial concerns, 85
Fishing, 65
Flare-up management plan, 176
Flare-ups, 175–178
Flexeril (cyclobenzaprine), 192
Flexibility, 76
Food
    enjoyment of, 65, 178
    and nutritional tiredness, 77–79
Fordyce, Bill, 172
Frequency, 119
Friends
    negative effects of, 6, 41–42
    and relaxation techniques, 64
    sharing with, 91–92. *See also*
        Communication
Frustration, 6, 82, 100

G

Gabapentin (Neurontin), 185
Gambling, 75, 122
Gardening, 35, 174
Gate-control theory of pain, 16–18, 22
Goals
    for behavioral change, 123
    and fatigue, 75
    mechanics of setting, 166–167
    for physical movement, 28, 37–40
    SMART, 121, 145, 146
Goodrich, Richelle E., 27
Grief, 134
Guided visualization, 61–62, 70–71
Guilt, 82, 100, 118

H

Headaches
    biofeedback for treatment of, 187
    online resources for, 204
    research on management of, 7
    unidentifiable causes of, 14
Heads Up podcast, 204
Health care provider shopping, 115–117
Health Experiences Research Group
        (Oxford University), 202
Health Talk website, 202
Heart problems, 57
Heart rate, 51
Heart surgery, 20
Heat therapy, 195
Help, 152–153
Hepburn, Audrey, 89
Hip replacement surgery, 15, 20
Hobbies, 35, 61, 173
Home activities
    for communication, 105
    for increasing physical movement, 44–47
    for increasing relaxation, 68
    for management of fatigue, 87–88
    for management of stressful thoughts
        and feelings, 142–143
    overview, 23
    for pain management, 168–169
Home environment, 63–64
Housework, 35, 38
Humor, 103
Hypnosis, 189

I

Immune system changes, 56
Indifferent-type people, 100, 104
Infections, 56
Insurance, 14
Interdependence, 151
International Association for the Study of
        Pain, 203
International Pelvic Pain Society, 204–205
Internet resources, 173, 201–205
Interpersonal conflict, 127–128
Interstitial cystitis, 205
Isolation, 90–91

J

James, William, 127, 161
Jealousy, 118
Journaling, 84

K

Ketoprofen, 195
Klonopin (clonazepam), 192

Knee replacement surgery, 15, 20
Knowledge, 166

L

Lancey, R., 201
Laws of learning, 109, 114–115, 162–163
Learning, 109, 114–115, 154, 162–163
Libraries, 173
Lidocaine patch, 195
Lidoderm, 195
Listening, 103
Literature, 173
Lorazepam (Ativan), 192
Love, 150–151
Lyrica (pregabalin), 185

M

Magnetic resonance images (MRIs), 14
Maintenance of change, 171–180
    home activities for, 180
    and managing flare-ups, 175–178
    and principles of pain management,
        171–175
Manual therapy, 193
Marijuana, 187–188
Massage, 65, 178, 190
Medicare, 85
Medication. *See also specific headings*
    antianxiety, 56–57
    effectiveness of, 19–20
    side effects of, 55
Meditation, 61, 80, 190, 194
Memory, 54, 162
Mental imagery, 57
Methocarbamol (Robaxin), 192
Migraine Monitor App, 204
Migraines, 13, 14, 204
Milnacipran (Savella), 186
Mindfulness techniques, 190
Mind reading (thinking error), 131, 179
Mitochondria, 73
Mixed agent drugs, 190–191
Mobile resources, 201–205
Mobility, 28
Model building, 173
Morphine, 77
Motivation, 165, 167
Movies, 63, 84
MRIs (magnetic resonance images), 14
Murphy's Law, 175
Muscle relaxants, 192–193
Muscle tension
    and fatigue, 81
    and relaxation techniques, 66, 67
    from stress, 51, 52
Muscle weakness, 29–30, 38

Musculoskeletal pain, 28
Music, 61, 173, 178
"Must" statements, 130, 135–137

N

Naps, 81
National Fibromyalgia and Chronic Pain
    Association, 203
National Headache Foundation, 204
Nature, 65, 84, 174
Negative thinking, 131
Nerve blocks, 191
Neurontin (gabapentin), 185
Neuropathic pain, 28
Niebuhr, Rheinhold, 11
Nonassertion, 98
N1-Headache app, 204
Nonsteroidal anti-inflammatory drugs
    (NSAIDs), 184–185, 195
Nutritional tiredness, 77–79

O

Occupational therapy, 192
Opioids
    dependence on, 3
    effectiveness of, 3–4
    function of, 184, 185
    and reinforcement, 120
Organ transplants, 5
Osteoarthritis, 195
Osteopaths, 193
Ouchie (app), 202
"Ought" statements, 130
Overgeneralization (thinking error), 131

P

Pacing (timing of behavior), 35–42, 81–82
Pain, 11–25
    behavior related to, 134
    common myths about, 17–21
    common treatments for, 183–196
    definitions of chronic, 12–15
    home activities for making sense of, 23
    questions to consider with, 22
    reality of, 15–17
Pain clinics, 191
Pain Concern website, 202
Pain Connection, 202
Pain-denying people, 99–100, 104
Pain gate
    factors in, 129, 131, 142, 162, 179
    overview, 16–18, 22
Pain management, 161–169. *See also specific*
        headings
    goal setting for, 166–167
    home activities for, 168–169

and power to change, 163–166
    questions to consider with, 168
    time orientation for, 162–163
Pain self-assessment, 24–25, 106–107,
        181–182
Pain signaling
    and gate-control theory, 16–18, 22
    reliability of, 13–14, 17, 178
Painting, 84, 173
Paracetamol, 184–185
Parenting, 112
Partners, 101–103
Passive coping, 28
Passivity, 122, 129, 148
Patient assistance programs, 85
Pavlov, Ivan, 113
Peanuts (cartoon), 6
Pelvic pain, 13, 204–205
Pelvic Pain Support Network, 205
Perfectionism, 149
Peripheral neuropathy, 193
Personality, 164
Pets, 178
Phantom limb pain, 15, 193
Pharmaceutical companies, 85
Physical movement, 27–47
    and balance, 30–31
    building strength with, 33–35
    conscientious, 31–32
    enjoyment of, 32–33
    and fatigue, 76, 79
    home activities for, 44–47
    importance of, 20
    pacing yourself with, 35–42
    and physical therapy, 192
    as principle of pain management,
        175–178
    questions to consider with, 43–44
    and weakened muscles, 29–30
Physical therapy, 192
Physical tiredness, 75–77
Pilates, 36, 192
Pilates, Joseph, 192
Poetry, 166
Polarized thinking, 130
Political involvement, 174
Portion size, 79
Positive in Pain group, 202
Postherpetic neuralgia, 193
Postural yoga, 194
Posture, 75
Prayer, 61
Predictability, 119
Pregabalin (Lyrica), 185
Present orientation, 156
Price, Reynolds, 156
Priorities, 84–85
Problem-solving, 28, 154–157
Progressive muscle relaxation, 58, 68–69

Progress tracking
   and function of, 167
   for physical movement, 40–41, 43–47
   and reinforcement, 121
Protective-type people, 99, 100, 104

Q

Quality time, 92
Quilting, 84, 166, 173

R

Radiculitis, 193
Reading, 61, 63, 84
Realism, 156
Realistic thinking, 132
Recovery, 33
Referred pain, 15, 196
Rehabilitation programs, 191
Reinforcement
   for behavioral change, 110–112,
     118–122
   types of consequences in, 114
Rejection, 100
Relapse prevention, 176
Relationships, 89. *See also* Communication
Relaxation techniques, 49–71
   and attention, 173
   benefits of, 65–66
   and conserving energy, 52
   and energy balance, 50–51
   home activities for, 68
   and indicators of stress, 51–56
   for maintenance of change, 172
   practicing of, 179
   questions to consider with, 67–68
   scripts for, 68–71
   tracking of, 167
   types of, 56–65
Relief website, 203
Religious materials, 61
Resentment, 100
Resilience, 117, 145, 157
Respect, 97, 98, 147
Respectful-type people, 100–101, 104
Rest
   and behavioral change, 120, 123
   and fatigue, 73
   and physical movement, 28, 38–39, 42–43
   and self-confidence, 146
Rewards (reinforcement), 119–122
Risk-taking, 156
Robaxin (methocarbamol), 192
Romanticism, 102

S

Sadness, 82, 118, 134
Safety, 91, 138

Sanchez, Roselyn, 171
Savella (milnacipran), 186
SCS (spinal cord stimulation), 193
Security, 91
Sedatives, 192–193
Selective serotonin and norepinephrine
   reuptake inhibitors (SSNRIs), 186
Self-acceptance, 147–149
Self-compassion, 146–149
Self-confidence, 145–159
   challenges to, 132
   development of, 80, 138
   and loving yourself, 149–154
   practicing of, 134
   problem-solving with, 154–157
   and self-compassion, 146–149
Self-expectations, 82–84, 135–137
Self-love, 150
Self-talk, 127
Sensory focus, 61–63
Sensory overload, 53
Serenity Prayer, 11, 12, 85, 134, 148, 179
Setbacks, 42, 43
Sewing, 84, 173
Sexual intercourse, 101
Shame, 6, 82, 100, 118
"Should" statements, 130, 135–137
Shyness, 134
Sleep. *See also* Fatigue
   difficulties with, 55
   and faulty thinking, 132
   importance of, 179
   improvement in quality of, 79–81
   and stress, 49
Sleeping pills, 122, 192–193
SMART (specific, measurable, achievable,
   relevant, timely) goals
   and autonomy, 156
   and motivation, 165
   overview, 121, 127
   and self-confidence, 145, 146
Smoking, 121, 123, 164
Snacking, 77
Social media, 61
Social outings, 54, 173–174
Specific, measurable, achievable, relevant,
   timely goals. *See* SMART goals
Spinal cord damage, 15
Spinal cord stimulation (SCS), 193
Spinal manipulations, 193
Spine Universe website, 203
Spirituality, 61
Sports, 166
SSNRIs (selective serotonin and
   norepinephrine reuptake
   inhibitors), 186
Stamina, 36
State health insurance assistance
   programs, 85

Stimulants, 55, 80
Stomach problems, 55–56
Strength, 76
Stress, 51–56. *See also* Relaxation
    techniques
Stressful thoughts and feelings, 127–143
    ABCD model for management of,
        138–141
    and behaving differently, 133–134
    home activities for management of,
        142–143
    questions to consider with, 142
    and self-expectations, 135–137
    and stopping at the right time, 137–138
    and thinking differently, 127–132
Stretching exercises, 36
Success, 157
Suffering, 177–178
Surgeries. *See also specific headings*
    for cancer, 14
    emotional effects of, 162
    expected healing for, 13
    and gate-control theory of pain, 17
    for pain management, 193–194
    prevalence of, 19
Swimming, 36
Systematic muscle relaxation, 58, 68–69

T

Tai chi, 194
Telephone conversations, 61
Television, 63, 84, 178
TENS (transcutaneous electrical nerve
    stimulation), 195–196
Tension headaches, 14
Tetrahydrocannabinol (THC), 187–188
Thermal therapies, 195
Thinking errors, 129–131
Timers, 34, 81
Timing, 119
Tolstoy, Leo, 16
Topamax (Trileptal), 185
Topical agents, 195
Tramadol (Ultram), 190–191
Tranquilizers, 192–193
Transcutaneous electrical nerve stimulation
    (TENS), 195–196
Travel, 54, 84
Treadmills, 36
Treatments for chronic pain, 183–196.
    See also specific headings
Trigger point injections, 196
Trileptal (Topamax), 185

U

Ultrasound stimulation, 196
Uncertainty, 54
Uniqueness, 149–150
U.S. National Institutes of Health, 184
U.S. Pain Foundation, 202

V

Valium (diazepam), 192
Varghese, E., 201
Venlafaxine (Effexor), 186
Video games, 61
Visualization techniques, 61–62, 70–71
Volunteer work, 35, 173
Vulvar pain, 205

W

Walking activities
    establishing baseline for, 37
    and physical movement, 31–32
    and treadmills, 36
Water activity, 31
Water aerobics, 41
Weather, 40, 85, 176
Weight gain, 56, 76, 78
Weights
    and pacing, 36, 40
    weekly goals for working with, 38
Whiplash
    and fatigue, 76
    treatments for, 193
    and unidentifiable causes of pain, 14
A Whole New Life (Price), 156
Wired (magazine), 201
Women's Pelvic Health podcast, 204
Woodworking, 173

X

X-rays, 14

Y

Yoga, 36, 59, 194
Yoo, I., 201
Yo-yo dieting, 34

Z

Zhao, P., 201
Zostrix, 195

ABOUT THE AUTHORS

Dennis C. Turk, PhD, has been involved in the assessment and treatment of people with various chronic pain conditions for over 30 years. He is currently the John and Emma Bonica Endowed Chair in Anesthesiology and Pain Research and a professor of anesthesiology and pain medicine at the University of Washington in Seattle. He is also currently associate director of Analgesic, Anesthetic, and Addiction Clinical Trial Translations, Innovations, Opportunities, and Networks, a public–private partnership supported by the U.S. Food and Drug Administration; and editor-in-chief of *The Clinical Journal of Pain*. He is a past president of the American Pain Society. Dr. Turk has published over 700 scientific journal articles and book chapters related to all aspects of pain, the conduct of clinical trials, and clinical practice. In addition, he has written or edited 33 volumes devoted to pain and coping and adaptation, most recently *Psychological Approaches to Pain Management: A Practitioner's Handbook* (3rd ed.) and *Whiplash Injury: Perspectives on the Development of Chronic Pain*. Dr. Turk's research has been supported by the National Institutes of Health, the U.S. Food and Drug Administration, the National Center for Health Statistics, the Patient-Centered Outcomes Research Institute, and several private foundations.

Frits Winter, PhD, received his doctoral degree in clinical psychology in 1992. His research focused on the effectiveness of self-help programs for chronic pain. He is a pioneer in developing therapy programs for chronic pain in the Netherlands. From 1983 to 2002, Dr. Winter was head of the Pain Division in the Roessingh Rehabilitation Center in Enschede, Netherlands. From a modest beginning, the department grew under his leadership to a pain clinic with

350 inpatients and 1,200 outpatients per year. He has been awarded for his excellent work with the Golden Roessingh Spell of Honor. Dr. Winter was president of the Dutch chapter of the International Association for the Study of Pain from 1996 to 2002. In 2002, he opened Medisch Centrum Winter, a treatment center for pain, stress, and burnout, in Veldhoven near Eindhoven, Netherlands. Dr. Winter is the author of several self-help books on the topics of pain, anxiety, fatigue, and memory. More than 60,000 copies of his first book about pain have been sold. He has been working with Dr. Turk for over 20 years, and together they published the first edition of *The Pain Survival Guide* in 2006.